10 Years Weight Loss,

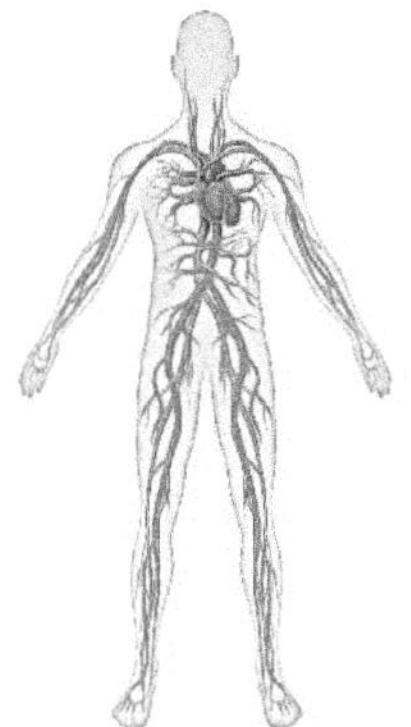

10 Years Vegetarian,

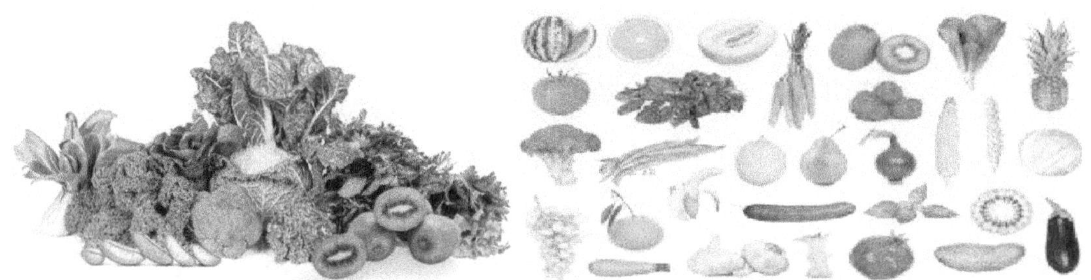

& 10 Years Organic

Part 2

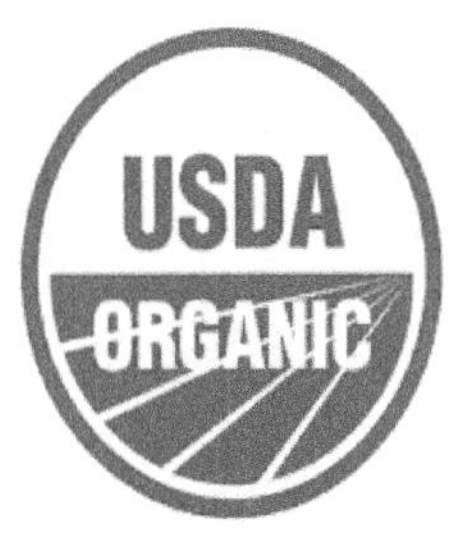

By Mary Hubbard

Nutrition Goals Completed 8/31/2020

8/31/2012	8 YEARS CONSECUTIVE WEIGHT LOSS
8/31/2012	2,923 DAYS CONSECUTIVE WEIGHT LOSS
1/01/2013	7 YEARS, 8 MONTHS CONSECUTIVE YEARS NO MEATS, NO DESERTS, NO SODA (CARBONATED BEVERAGES), NO CAFFEINE, NO CANDY, AND REDUCED SUGAR INTAKE TO 10 GRAMS OR LESS PER SERVING FOR SINGLE EDIBLE FOOD ITEMS
5/01/2013	OVER 7 CONSECUTIVE YEARS CONSUMING ONLY CERTIFIED ORGANIC AND OR ALL NATURAL VITAMINS, SUPPLEMENTS, AND OR HERBS (VITAMINS, MINERALS, AND HERBS)
6/01/2013	OVER 7 CONSECUTIVE YEARS NO CONSUMPTION OF MICROWAVE HEATED FOODS OR BEVERAGES
6/15/2013	OVER 7 CONSECUTIVE YEARS CONSISTENTLY SHOPPING @ WHOLE FOODS ON A WEEKLY BASIS
7/01/2013	OVER 7 CONSECUTIVE YEARS CONSUMING ORGANIC CERTIFIED AND OR FOODS WITH ORGANIC INGREDIENTS AND BEVERAGES (EXCEPT FOR WATER)
4/01/2014	ALMOST 6 ½ CONSECUTIVE YEARS GLUTEN-FREE, SOY-FREE, AND REDUCED FRIED FOOD INTAKE
4/01/2014	OVER 6 CONSECUTIVE YEARS, NO FOOD CONSUMPTION BETWEEN THE HOURS OF 6:00 P.M. AND 6:00 A.M.
2/10/2015	OVER 5 ½ CONSECUTIVE YEARS, NO FRIED FOOD INTAKE
7/15/2016	OVER 3 ½ CONSECUTIVE YEARS OF DAILY LIMITED SATURATED FAT CONSUMPTION (WITH THE EXCEPTION OF AVOCADOS, CASHEWS, NUTS, ETC.) NO LIMIT OF DAILY UNSATURATED FAT INTAKE
1/01/2017	OVER 3 ½ YEARS OF DAILY CONSUMPTION OF FRESH VEGETABLES AND FRUITS (9-13 SERVINGS RECOMMENDED AMOUNT) AND DRINKING DAILY RECOMMENDED AMOUNT OF WATER OR MORE

Nutrition Goals Completed 12/31/2022

8/31/2012   10 YEARS 4 MONTHS CONSECUTIVE WEIGHT LOSS

8/31/2012   3,774 DAYS CONSECUTIVE WEIGHT LOSS

1/01/2013   10 YEARS CONSECUTIVE YEARS NO MEATS, NO DESERTS, NO CARBONATED BEVERAGES, NO CAFFEINE, NO CANDY, AND REDUCED SUGAR INTAKE TO 10 GRAMS OR LESS PER SERVING FOR SINGLE EDIBLE FOOD ITEMS

5/01/2013   OVER 9 ½ CONSECUTIVE YEARS CONSUMING ONLY CERTIFIED ORGANIC AND OR ALL NATURAL VITAMINS, SUPPLEMENTS, AND OR HERBS (VITAMINS, MINERALS, AND HERBS)

6/01/2013   9 ½ CONSECUTIVE YEARS OF NO CONSUMPTION OF MICROWAVE-HEATED FOODS OR BEVERAGES

6/15/2013   9 ½ CONSECUTIVE YEARS CONSISTENTLY SHOPPING @ WHOLE FOODS ON A WEEKLY BASIS

7/01/2013   ALMOST 9 ½ CONSECUTIVE YEARS CONSUMING ORGANIC CERTIFIED AND OR FOODS WITH ORGANIC INGREDIENTS AND BEVERAGES (EXCEPT FOR WATER)

4/01/2014   ALMOST 9 CONSECUTIVE YEARS GLUTEN-FREE, SOY-FREE, AND REDUCED FRIED FOOD INTAKE

4/01/2014   ALMOST 9 CONSECUTIVE YEARS OF NO FOOD CONSUMPTION BETWEEN THE HOURS OF 6:00 P.M. AND 6:00 A.M.

2/10/2015   ALMOST 8 CONSECUTIVE YEARS OF NO FRIED FOOD INTAKE

7/15/2016   NEARLY 6 ½ CONSECUTIVE YEARS OF DAILY LIMITED SATURATED FAT CONSUMPTION (WITH THE EXCEPTION OF AVOCADOS, CASHEWS, NUTS, ETC.) NO LIMIT OF DAILY UNSATURATED FAT INTAKE

1/01/2017   6 YEARS OF DAILY CONSUMPTION OF FRESH VEGETABLES AND FRUITS (9-13 SERVINGS RECOMMENDED AMOUNT) AND DRINKING DAILY RECOMMENDED AMOUNT OF WATER OR MORE ON AVERAGE

11/16/2020   OVER 2 YEARS, CONSISTENTLY EXERCISING SEVERAL TIMES PER WEEK
              ON AVERAGE

3/15/2021   ALMOST 2 YEARS ZERO TO LOW GLYCEMIC INDEX FOODS, HIGH FIBER,
              & HIGH PROTEIN FOOD CONSUMPTION

9/15/2021   ALMOST 1 ½ YEARS INCLUDING RAW ORGANIC ROOIBOS TEA AND OR
              ORGANIC ANTIOXIDANT CAFFEINE FREE TEA IN MY ORGANIC HOMEMADE
              FRUIT & VEGETABLE JUICE

Nutrition Goals 12/31/2023

8/31/2012   11 YEARS 4 MONTHS CONSECUTIVE WEIGHT LOSS

8/31/2012   4,139 DAYS CONSECUTIVE WEIGHT LOSS

1/01/2013   11 YEARS CONSECUTIVE YEARS NO MEATS, NO DESERTS, NO SODA
              (CARBONATED BEVERAGES), NO CAFFEINE, NO CANDY, AND REDUCED
              SUGAR INTAKE TO 10 GRAMS OR LESS PER SERVING FOR SINGLE EDIBLE
              FOOD ITEMS

5/01/2013   OVER 10 ½ CONSECUTIVE YEARS CONSUMING ONLY CERTIFIED ORGANIC
              AND OR ALL NATURAL VITAMINS, SUPPLEMENTS, AND OR HERBS
              (VITAMINS, MINERALS, AND HERBS)

6/01/2013   10 ½ CONSECUTIVE YEARS OF NO CONSUMPTION OF MICROWAVE-HEATED
              FOODS OR BEVERAGES

6/15/2013   10 ½ CONSECUTIVE YEARS CONSISTENTLY SHOPPING @ WHOLE FOODS ON
              A WEEKLY BASIS

7/01/2013   ALMOST 10 ½ CONSECUTIVE YEARS CONSUMING ORGANIC CERTIFIED AND
              OR FOODS WITH ORGANIC INGREDIENTS AND BEVERAGES (EXCEPT FOR
              WATER)

4/01/2014   ALMOST 10 CONSECUTIVE YEARS GLUTEN-FREE, SOY-FREE, AND
              REDUCED FRIED FOOD INTAKE

4/01/2014   ALMOST 10 CONSECUTIVE YEARS NO FOOD CONSUMPTION BETWEEN THE
              HOURS OF 6:00 P.M. AND 6:00 A.M.

2/10/2015	ALMOST 9 CONSECUTIVE YEARS NO FRIED FOOD INTAKE
7/15/2016	NEARLY 8 ½ CONSECUTIVE YEARS OF DAILY LIMITED SATURATED FAT CONSUMPTION (WITH THE EXCEPTION OF AVOCADOS, CASHEWS, NUTS, ETC.) NO LIMIT OF DAILY UNSATURATED FAT INTAKE
1/01/2017	7 YEARS OF CONSUMPTION OF VEGETABLES AND FRUITS (5 OR MORE SERVINGS) AND DRINKING DAILY RECOMMENDED AMOUNT OF WATER OR MORE (Mondays – Fridays)
11/16/2020	OVER 3 YEARS CONSISTENTLY EXERCISING SEVERAL TIMES PER WEEK ON AVERAGE
3/15/2021	ALMOST 3 YEARS ZERO TO LOW GLYCEMIC INDEX FOODS, HIGH FIBER, & HIGH PROTEIN FOOD CONSUMPTION
9/15/2021	ALMOST 2 ½ YEARS CONSUMPTION OF RAW ORGANIC ROOIBOS TEA AND OR ORGANIC ANTIOXIDANT CAFFEINE FREE TEA

Nutrition Goals 12/31/2024

8/31/2012	12 YEARS CONSECUTIVE WEIGHT LOSS
8/31/2012	4,505 DAYS CONSECUTIVE WEIGHT LOSS
1/01/2013	12 YEARS CONSECUTIVE YEARS NO MEATS, NO DESERTS, NO SODA (CARBONATED BEVERAGES), NO CAFFEINE, NO CANDY, AND REDUCED SUGAR INTAKE TO 10 GRAMS OR LESS PER SERVING FOR SINGLE EDIBLE FOOD ITEMS
5/01/2013	OVER 11 ½ CONSECUTIVE YEARS CONSUMING ONLY CERTIFIED ORGANIC AND OR ALL NATURAL VITAMINS, SUPPLEMENTS, AND OR HERBS (VITAMINS, MINERALS, AND HERBS)
6/01/2013	11 ½ CONSECUTIVE YEARS NO CONSUMPTION OF MICROWAVE HEATED FOODS OR BEVERAGES
6/15/2013	11 ½ CONSECUTIVE YEARS CONSISTENTLY SHOPPING @ WHOLE FOODS ON A WEEKLY BASIS

7/01/2013	ALMOST 11 ½ CONSECUTIVE YEARS CONSUMING ORGANIC CERTIFIED AND OR FOODS WITH ORGANIC INGREDIENTS AND BEVERAGES (EXCEPT FOR WATER)
4/01/2014	ALMOST 11 CONSECUTIVE YEARS OF GLUTEN-FREE, SOY-FREE, AND REDUCED FRIED FOOD INTAKE
4/01/2014	ALMOST 11 CONSECUTIVE YEARS OF NO FOOD CONSUMPTION BETWEEN THE HOURS OF 6:00 P.M. AND 6:00 A.M.
2/10/2015	ALMOST 10 CONSECUTIVE YEARS OF NO FRIED FOOD INTAKE
7/15/2016	NEARLY 9 ½ CONSECUTIVE YEARS OF DAILY LIMITED SATURATED FAT CONSUMPTION (WITH THE EXCEPTION OF AVOCADOS, CASHEWS, NUTS, ETC.) NO LIMIT OF DAILY UNSATURATED FAT INTAKE
1/01/2017	7 YEARS OF CONSUMPTION OF VEGETABLES AND FRUITS (5 OR MORE SERVINGS) AND DRINKING DAILY RECOMMENDED AMOUNT OF WATER OR MORE (Mondays – Fridays)
11/16/2020	OVER 4 YEARS, CONSISTENTLY EXERCISING SEVERAL TIMES PER WEEK ON AVERAGE
3/15/2021	ALMOST 4 YEARS ZERO TO LOW GLYCEMIC INDEX FOODS, HIGH FIBER, & HIGH PROTEIN FOOD CONSUMPTION
9/15/2021	ALMOST 2 ½ YEARS OF CONSUMPTION OF RAW ORGANIC ROOIBOS TEA AND OR ORGANIC ANTIOXIDANT CAFFEINE-FREE TEA

Overall Nutritional & Exercise Goals 12/31/2023

- 12 Years Total Nutritional Practices
- (1 year several days per week then 11 years everyday),
- Over 11 Years Consecutive Weight Loss,
- 11 Years Consecutive Vegetarian,
- 10 ½ Years Consistently Shopping @ Whole Foods,
- 10 ½ Years Consecutive Consumption of Organic Foods, &
- 3 Years Consistent Exercise

Overall Nutritional & Exercise Goals 12/31/2024

- 13 Years Total Nutritional Practices
- (1 year several days per week then 12 years everyday),
- Over 12 Years Consecutive Weight Loss,
- 12 Years Consecutive Vegetarian,
- 11 ½ Years Consistently Shopping @ Whole Foods,
- 11 ½ Years Consecutive Consumption of Organic Foods, &
- 4 Years Consistent Exercise

Introduction

I previously wrote about my personal nutritional journey in my prior book Titled 7 Years Weight Loss, 7 Years Vegetarian, and 7 Years Organic. This book is intended to provide readers with updates on my nutritional practices.

This book provides helpful nutritional tips and an understanding of bodily and physiological functions. This book depicts the total picture of nutrition, not just one facet. This book explains how nutrition impacts arthritis, DNA, hormones, cancer, cholesterol and heart disease, the immune system, infertility, the change of life, inflammation, protecting our bodies against the harmful effects of pollution, the lungs and respiratory system, and so much more. This book also discusses the roles of antioxidants, amino acids, cholesterol, healthy fats, salt, fiber, protein, hydration, and so much more.

In a lot of instances, nutrition can function as a medicine. More importantly, nutrition can prevent many ailments and diseases.

This book discusses the consistency of healthy nutritional habits, which is very important. In order for me to continue to be consistent, I developed new eating patterns.

The content of this book is comprised of my personal life experiences and lots of research. I have read over 500 articles and journals written by national associations and agencies, leading doctors and physicians, leading certified dietitians, leading nutritionists, and leading natural and wellness experts so that I can write this book in addition to all of the health and nutrition-related articles I read during this journey.

I want to thank you for getting this book. I hope you have as much fun reading this book as I did writing it.

Contents

Chapter 1

Vegan versus Vegetarian

I chose to become a vegetarian. People choose to become vegetarians or vegans for different reasons. Some people are vehemently against exploitation of animals. They perceive the slaughter of animals as cruel and inhumane. Some believe meat and or dairy products offers little to no nutritional value. I chose to become a vegetarian, because it was easier for me to abstain from unhealthy food groups when I said no to meat. Years ago, during my undergraduate studies, I used to be a vegetarian. It lasted for almost a year. This time it is permanent.

The Vegetarian Society defines a vegetarian as follows:

"A vegetarian is someone who lives on a diet of pulses, legumes, nuts, seeds, vegetables, fruits, fungi, algae, yeast and/or some other non-animal-based foods (e.g. salt) with, or without, dairy products, honey and/or eggs. A vegetarian does not eat foods that consist of or have been produced with the aid of products consisting of or created from, any part of the body of a living or dead animal. This includes meat, poultry, fish, shellfish*, insects, by-products of slaughter or any food made with processing aids created from these."

There are different types of vegetarian:

1. Lacto-ovo-vegetarians eat both dairy products and eggs; this is the most common type of vegetarian diet.

2. Lacto-vegetarians eat dairy products but avoid eggs.

3. Ovo-vegetarian. Eats eggs but not dairy products.

4. Vegans do not eat dairy products, eggs, or any other products which are derived from animals.

I am a lacto-ovo-vegetarian.

Veganism is a way of living which seeks to exclude as far as possible and practicable, all forms of exploitation of, and cruelty to, animals for food, clothing or any other purpose. All vegans adhere to a plant-based diet avoiding all animal foods such as meat (including fish, shellfish, and insects) diary, eggs, honey leather, fur, and any products tested on animals.

There are distinctive differences between vegans and vegetarians. A vegetarian excludes meat, poultry, and seafood from their diet. Some vegetarians also exclude dairy, some don't, and some may consume eggs. Likewise, vegans avoid meat, poultry, and seafood, but they also take it a step further by eliminating all animal products from their diet. This includes any type of animal milk and eggs. Vegans avoid foods produced using animals or animal products in any way, including honey. Many vegans also avoid household products, clothing, or other items made from animal products or tested on animals.Undoubtedly, there is a modern conflict between vegans and vegetarians. The conflict is that vegetarians are not true vegetarians or true vegetarians does not exist anymore if or because of their consumption of dairy products.

There are different types of vegetarians. A person's decision or choice to become a vegetarian instead of a vegan is not necessarily indicative of less nutritional discipline and or will power.

Although I am not professional medical practitioner, my hypothesis is that there are some health and or nutritional benefits with regard to consuming dairy products. Vegetarians who consume dairy products but do not eat meat are possibly benefiting from the amino acids from dairy products in comparison to plant-based proteins another vegan suggested sources of proteins which are subsequently converted into glucose or sugar during the digestion process. This benefit can also be correlated to increased energy. In place of caffeine, I regularly consume the B-12 supplements and healthy diary protein foods.

Please don't get me wrong. The purpose or the intent of this chapter is not to bash or criticize vegans or those who disregard vegetarians. The intended purpose of this chapter is to point out the difference between vegans and vegetarians, who should be able to peacefully coexist.

Chapter 2

No Meats, Limited Sugar, and No Caffeine

I am going to tell on myself. I used to be a "potato-chip" person. Although there is technically not a lot of sugar content in potatoes, they turn into sugar when they are digested. Potatoes are a form of starch. Starch or amylum is a polymeric carbohydrate consisting of a large amounts of glucose units, which are joined by glycosidic bonds. This polysaccharide is produced by most green plants as energy storage. It is the most common carbohydrate in human diets and is contained in large amounts in staple foods like potatoes, wheat, maize (corn), rice, and cassava.

It can be surprising to find out that potatoes are generally high on the glycemic index (GI), which rates how much certain foods raise your blood glucose. Plus, most people associate blood sugar with foods that contain sugar. How is it that a potato has a higher GI than white sugar? It's all about the starch and how it converts to glucose in your body. Since the starch in potatoes is rapidly digested, the glycemic index of potatoes can be almost as high as that of glucose alone. The glycemic index of glucose is 100 points where potatoes are usually listed as being in the high 80s or low 90s. Carbohydrates are also converted into sugar when digested. You may want to refer to the Carbohydrates section of chapter 1 for the definition and examples of refined, simple carbohydrates and complex carbohydrates.

I am not concerned with the amount of carbohydrates I consume or "carb counting", salt intake, or cholesterol intake. I am more concerned with the amount of sugar I consume. Too often people vilify salt and cholesterol. However, salt and cholesterol play important roles in our bodies. People often argue the amount of salt eaten has a direct effect on blood pressure. They argue salt makes your body hold on to water. If you eat too much salt, water is stored in your body. This results in an elevated blood pressure. The more salt eaten, the higher your blood pressure will be. Higher blood pressure creates a strain on your heart, arteries, kidneys, and brain. This can result in heart attacks, strokes, dementia, and kidney disease. They say eating too much salt hinders blood pressure medicines including diuretics from working as well as they could.

Sodium is an essential nutrient but is something that the body cannot produce itself. It plays a vital role in the regulation of many bodily functions and is contained in body fluids that transport oxygen and nutrients. Water serves as the primary component of the fluids that circulate in your body. Depending on your age and muscle mass, water makes up anywhere from 45 to 75 percent of your body weight. Your body possesses two main fluid compartments: intracellular fluid is inside your cells, and extracellular fluid circulates outside cells. Salt, an electrolyte, plays a major role in extracellular fluids as the most abundant ion group. Your kidneys play a critical part in maintaining sodium and water balance. The balance of water and sodium is critical to your health. Salt is essential in maintaining the body's overall fluid balance. To survive everyone needs to consume sodium regularly. It is a principal component of a person's internal environment – the extracellular fluid. Nutrients reach your body's cells through these fluids. Sodium facilitates many bodily functions including fluid volume and acid-base balance.

The human body can't live without some sodium. In addition to maintaining blood pressure, sodium is needed for proper function of your nerves, muscles and other body tissues. It's needed to transmit nerve impulses, contract and relax muscle fibers (including those in the heart and blood vessels), and maintain a proper fluid balance. Problems occur when too much or not enough sodium is in your body. Diuretic medicines, drinking too much water, excessive sweating, heart failure and kidney disease, among other conditions, can disrupt the balance of sodium to water. An imbalance can cause symptoms such as fatigue, headache and muscle spasms. Sodium enables the transmission of nerve impulses around the body. It is an electrolyte, like Potassium, Calcium and Magnesium; it regulates the electrical charges moving in and out of the cells in the body. It controls your taste, smell and tactile processes. The presence of sodium ions is essential for the contraction of muscles, including that largest and most important muscle, the heart. It is fundamental to the operation of signals to and from the brain. Without sufficient sodium your senses would be dulled and your nerves would not function. When sodium is in short supply, a host of chemical and hormonal messages signal the kidneys and sweat glands to hold onto water and conserve sodium.

An adult human body contains about 250g of salt and any excess is naturally excreted by the body. When you get more sodium than you need, the kidneys flush out the excess by making more, or saltier, urine. If they can't get rid of enough sodium, though, it accumulates in the fluid between cells. Water inevitably follows sodium, and as the volume of this fluid increases, so does the volume of blood. This means more work for the heart and more pressure on blood vessels. Over time, this can stiffen blood vessels, leading to high blood pressure, heart attack, or stroke. It can also lead to heart failure. There is also some evidence that salt can directly affect the heart, aorta, and kidneys without necessarily increasing blood pressure. Some people are exquisitely sensitive to salt "" their blood pressure rises and falls as a direct result of how much salt they get. Others don't seem to be affected at all. Unfortunately, there isn't an easy test to determine who is salt-sensitive. While your body's natural checks and balances help it adapt to varying sodium intakes, you'll help your body out if you limit the amount of sodium you consume in your diet. Too much sodium constantly "strains" your system, and can lead to high blood pressure, poorer bone health and more. Keep your sodium intake lower than 2,300 milligrams daily, or 1,500 milligrams if you're at risk of high blood pressure or heart disease.

Most people think of cholesterol in a negative way. However, cholesterol actually plays a very important role in the functioning of the body. According to The Mayo Clinic, cholesterol is found in every cell in our body and without it our bodies would not function properly. Understanding why it is there and the purpose it serves is something everyone should be aware of. Cholesterol is a waxy, fat-like substance that's found in all the cells in your body. Your body needs some cholesterol to make hormones, vitamin D, and substances that help you digest foods. Your body makes all the cholesterol it needs. Cholesterol is also found in foods from animal sources, such as egg yolks, meat, and cheese. Cholesterol in your body comes from two main sources: your liver and your diet. Your liver, other organs, and other cells in your body produce about 75 percent of the cholesterol in your blood. The other 25 percent of cholesterol in your body is affected by the foods you eat. As you take in more cholesterol, your liver compensates by reducing its own production of cholesterol and removing excess cholesterol. Some experts believe there is no need to eat foods high in cholesterol. They believe the body is very good at making its own cholesterol - you don't need to help it along. They believe you don't need to eat foods that contain cholesterol. Your body can produce all the cholesterol it needs.

Cholesterol is produced by the liver and also made by most cells in the body. It is carried around in the blood by little 'couriers' called lipoproteins. Cholesterol builds the structure of cell membranes, make hormones like estrogen, testosterone and adrenal hormones, helps your metabolism work efficiently, for example, cholesterol is essential for your body to produce vitamin D, and helps the liver to produce bile acids, which help the body digest fat and absorb important nutrients.

Functions of Cholesterol:

1. Hormone Manufacturing: One of the most important jobs of cholesterol is to aide in the production of hormones. Cholesterol is stored in the adrenal glands, ovaries and the testes and is converted to steroid hormones. These steroid hormones perform other vital duties to help the body function properly. Without steroid hormones we will have malfunctions with weight, sex, digestion, bone health and mental status.
2. Digestion: Cholesterol plays an important role in our body's digestion. Cholesterol is used to help the liver create bile which aids us in digesting the food that we eat. Without the bile our bodies are unable to properly digest foods, especially fats. When the fat goes undigested it can get into the bloodstream and cause additional problems such as blockages of the arteries and cause heart attacks and heart disease.
3. Building Blocks: Cholesterol is a structural component of cells. Cholesterol along with polar lipids make up the structure of each and every cell in our bodies. Cholesterol is there to basically provide a protective barrier. When the amount of cholesterol increases or

decreases, the cells are affected. This change can affect our ability to metabolize and produce energy. This can ultimately affect other aspects of our bodies' function such as food intake and digestion.

Skinny people can have high cholesterol. A study found that about a quarter of Americans who aren't overweight have some form of an unhealthy heart risk, like high cholesterol or high blood pressure. High cholesterol does not discriminate against body type, and body weight does not determine if a person suffers from high cholesterol or high triglycerides (a type of fat in the blood). People who appear to be thinner assume they are not at risk. Therefore [they] don't heed the appropriate steps to take toward a healthier lifestyle, which may lead to higher cholesterol and triglyceride levels, and, ultimately, heart disease. As mentioned above, our bodies naturally make cholesterol. So, if you have a genetic predisposition to high cholesterol, yours will likely be elevated no matter how much you weigh. The American Heart Association recommends sticking to 300 mg of cholesterol or less each day to protect heart health. If you have been diagnosed with high cholesterol, you are advised to stay below 200 mg daily. Please reference the Nutrition, Colon, Detoxing, Fiber, and Immune System section of chapter 1 for further discussion of cholesterol.

However, too much HDL (high density lipoproteins) can also increase your risk for a heart attack and possibly other medical complications.

Several years ago, I heard a rumor that melted cheese is unhealthy. This rumor suggested that it is unmelted cheese that contains the health benefits. Therefore, I decided to research this matter further. Although melting the cheese concentrates the calories and fat, it also concentrates the nutrition. One cup of melted cheddar provides 176 percent of the recommended dietary allowance for calcium, based on a 2,000-calorie diet. It also provides 125 percent for phosphorus, 49 percent for vitamin A, 54 percent for riboflavin, 48 percent for selenium, 51 percent for zinc and 34 percent for vitamin B-12. Melted cheese contains smaller amounts of additional vitamins and minerals, including 17 percent for magnesium, 10 percent for pantothenic acid, 11 percent for folate, 9 percent for vitamin B-6, 9 percent for vitamin K, 7 percent for vitamin D and 9 percent for iron. By melting cheese, you get more cheese per serving – and more of the calories and nutrients. You would be inclined to believe unmelted cheese is healthier for you.

Sugars are carbohydrates, which serve as the main energy source for the body (except for those on the ketones diet). There are many types of sugars. They occur both naturally and as ingredients in many foods. The most familiar sugar is sucrose. It is made of two simple sugars, fructose and glucose. Fruits and vegetables naturally contain fructose and glucose. Other sugars used in foods include invert sugar, corn syrup, high fructose corn syrup, honey, lactose (milk sugar) and other syrups. During digestion, all of these sugars except lactose break down into fructose and glucose. Lactose breaks down into glucose and galactose.

Sugars are a source of energy for the body. During intense physical activity, they are the main energy source. There are no nutritional differences among sugars. The body uses all types in the same way. During digestion, sugars such as sucrose and lactose and other carbohydrates such as starches break down into simple (or single) sugars. Simple sugars then travel through the blood stream to body cells. There they provide energy and help form proteins or are stored for future use. The brain and red blood cells can only use glucose for energy. During pregnancy, glucose also helps form cells and produce milk. The body can make its own glucose or get it from foods.

The glycemic index (GI) is a ranking of foods on a scale of 0-100 according to how much they raise blood sugar levels. High-GI foods are digested rapidly and raise blood sugar levels quickly whereas low GI foods are more slowly digested and produce a gradual raise in glucose and insulin levels in the blood. Products with sugar, corn syrup, molasses, and hidden sugars (ingredients ending in -ose) usually indicate a high-GI food. The less processed a product is, the lower the GI will be. These foods usually have more fiber, which helps to delay digestion and also contain more vitamins, minerals and cancer-fighting phytochemicals. Sugary beverages like pop, energy or sports drinks, & sweetened teas/coffees are considered high GI products. These drinks are high in calories so they can cause weight gain if consumed often. Better beverage choices include water, unsweetened tea, vegetable juices, and milk since they have a low GI and contain other nutrients. Remember to opt for whole fruits & vegetables as they offer more fiber, cause less of an increase in blood sugar, and help to control hunger better than juice forms.

A fast increase in blood sugar causes a rapid increase in insulin, which is the hormone responsible for allowing glucose to enter cells. High insulin levels cause glucose levels to quickly fall, which can then cause you to feel hungry again, prompting you to take in more calories. Consistently high insulin levels can also cause cells to become resistant to insulin, meaning glucose levels stay higher for longer periods. High glucose levels, overweight/obesity, and inactivity can all increase the risk for diabetes and heart disease. Research has linked diabetes and obesity to cancers of the liver, pancreas, endometrium, colon and rectum, and bladder.

According to the American Heart Association (AHA), the maximum amount of added sugars you should eat in a day are:

1.   Men: 150 calories per day (37.5 grams or 9 teaspoons)

2.   Women: 100 calories per day (25 grams or 6 teaspoons)

Sugar that occurs naturally in whole fruit, however, does not count toward the 25 grams. Health experts point out that the sugar in whole fruit is not associated with any adverse health effects, primarily because of how the fiber in the fruit slows down the body's absorption of the sugar. Fruit contains natural sugars, which are a mix of sucrose, fructose and glucose. Some experts believe fructose is only harmful in excess amounts, and not when it comes from fruit. Some experts believe it would be incredibly difficult to consume excessive amounts of fructose by eating whole fruits. On the other hand, some experts believe if you exercise regularly and aren't overweight, your body can deal with simple sugars just fine. You're not going to get diabetes or ruin your heart by eating a bit more sugar than necessary every day. We've all heard of yellow urine being indicative of higher sugar intake. I don't know how true this is. Once the blood sugar level gets higher than 180 mg/dl, the kidneys start to spill sugar into the urine. The higher the blood sugar, the more sugar comes out in the urine. If your kidneys are normal, this usually isn't a problem.

Excessive sugar intake can cause:

1. Can Cause Weight Gain:

Rates of obesity are rising worldwide and added sugar, especially from sugar-sweetened beverages, is thought to be one of the main culprits. Sugar-sweetened drinks like sodas, juices and sweet teas are loaded with fructose, a type of simple sugar. Consuming fructose increases your hunger and desire for food more than glucose, the main type of sugar found in starchy foods. Additionally, excessive fructose consumption may cause resistance to leptin, an important hormone that regulates hunger and tells your body to stop eating. In other words, sugary beverages don't curb your hunger, making it easy to quickly consume a high number of liquid calories. This can lead to weight gain. Research has consistently shown that people who drink sugary beverages, such as soda and juice, weigh more than people who don't. Also, drinking a lot of sugar-sweetened beverages is linked to an increased amount of visceral fat, a kind of deep belly fat associated with conditions like diabetes and heart disease.

2. May Increase Your Risk of Heart Disease:

High-sugar diets have been associated with an increased risk of many diseases, including heart disease, the number one cause of death worldwide. Evidence suggests that high-sugar diets can lead to obesity, inflammation and high triglyceride, blood sugar and blood pressure levels — all risk factors for heart disease. Additionally, consuming too much sugar, especially from sugar-sweetened drinks, has been linked to atherosclerosis, a disease characterized by fatty, artery-clogging deposits.

3. Has Been Linked to Acne:

A diet high in refined carbs, including sugary foods and drinks, has been associated with a higher risk of developing acne. Foods with a high glycemic index, such as processed sweets, raise your blood sugar more rapidly than foods with a lower glycemic index. Sugary foods quickly spike blood sugar and insulin levels, causing increased androgen secretion, oil production and inflammation, all of which play a role in acne development. Studies have shown that low-glycemic diets are associated with a reduced acne risk, while high-glycemic diets are linked to a greater risk. For example, a study in 2,300 teens demonstrated that those who frequently consumed added sugar had a 30% greater risk of developing acne. Also, many population studies have shown that rural communities that consume traditional, non-processed foods have almost non-existent rates of acne, compared to more urban, high-income areas. These findings coincide with the theory that diets high in processed, sugar-laden foods contribute to the development of acne.

2. Increases Your Risk of Diabetes:

The worldwide prevalence of diabetes has more than doubled over the past 30 years. Though there are many reasons for this, there is a clear link between excessive sugar consumption and diabetes risk. Obesity, which is often caused by consuming too much sugar, is considered the strongest risk factor for diabetes. What's more, prolonged high-sugar consumption drives resistance to insulin, a hormone produced by the pancreas that regulates blood sugar levels. Insulin resistance causes blood sugar levels to rise and strongly increases your risk of diabetes.

3. May Increase Your Risk of Cancer:

Eating excessive amounts of sugar may increase your risk of developing certain cancers. First, a diet rich in sugary foods and beverages can lead to obesity, which significantly raises your risk of cancer. Furthermore, diets high in sugar increase inflammation in your body and may cause insulin resistance, both of which increase cancer risk. A study in over 430,000 people found that added sugar consumption was positively associated with an increased risk of esophageal cancer, pleural cancer and cancer of the small intestine. Another study showed that women who consumed sweet buns and cookies more than three times per week were 1.42 times more likely to develop endometrial cancer than women who consumed these foods less than 0.5 times per week.

4. May Increase Your Risk of Depression:

While a healthy diet can help improve your mood, a diet high in added sugar and processed foods may increase your chances of developing depression. Consuming a lot of processed foods, including high-sugar products such as cakes and sugary drinks, has been associated with a higher risk of depression. Researchers believe that blood sugar swings, neurotransmitter dysregulation and inflammation may all be reasons for sugar's detrimental impact on mental health.

5. May Accelerate the Skin Aging Process:

Wrinkles are a natural sign of aging. They appear eventually, regardless of your health. However, poor food choices can worsen wrinkles and speed the skin aging process. Advanced glycation end products (AGEs) are compounds formed by reactions between sugar and protein in your body. They are suspected to play a key role in skin aging. Consuming a diet high in refined carbs and sugar leads to the production of AGEs, which may cause your skin to age prematurely. AGEs damage collagen and elastin, which are proteins that help the skin stretch and keep its youthful appearance. When collagen and elastin become damaged, the skin loses its firmness and begins to sag. In one study, women who consumed more carbs, including added sugars, had a more wrinkled appearance than women on a high-protein, lower-carb diet. The researchers concluded that a lower intake of carbs was associated with better skin-aging appearance.

6. Can Increase Cellular Aging:

Remember telomeres from chapter 1. Telomeres are structures found at the end of chromosomes, which are molecules that hold part or all of your genetic information. Telomeres act as protective caps, preventing chromosomes from deteriorating or fusing together. As you grow older, telomeres naturally shorten, which causes cells to age and malfunction. Although the shortening of telomeres is a normal part of aging, unhealthy lifestyle choices can speed up the process. Consuming high amounts of sugar has been shown to accelerate telomere shortening, which increases cellular aging. A study in 5,309 adults showed that regularly drinking sugar-sweetened beverages was associated with shorter telomere length and premature cellular aging.

7. Drains Your Energy:

Foods high in added sugar quickly spike blood sugar and insulin levels, leading to increased energy. However, this rise in energy levels is fleeting. Products that are loaded with sugar but lacking in protein, fiber or fat lead to a brief energy boost that's quickly followed by a sharp drop in blood sugar, often referred to as a crash. Having constant blood sugar swings can lead to major fluctuations in energy levels. To avoid this energy-draining cycle, choose carb sources that are low in added sugar and rich in fiber. Pairing carbs with protein or fat is another great way to keep your blood sugar and energy levels stable.

8. Can Lead to Fatty Liver:

A high intake of fructose has been consistently linked to an increased risk of fatty liver. Unlike glucose and other types of sugar, which are taken up by many cells throughout the body, fructose is almost exclusively broken down by the liver. In the liver, fructose is converted into energy or stored as glycogen. However, the liver can only store so much glycogen before excess amounts are turned into fat. Large amounts of added sugar in the form of fructose overload your liver, leading to non-alcoholic fatty liver disease (NAFLD), a condition characterized by excessive fat buildup in the liver.

9. Other Health Risks:

Research shows that too much added sugar can:

a. Increase kidney disease risk: Having consistently high blood sugar levels can cause damage to the delicate blood vessels in your kidneys. This can lead to an increased risk of kidney disease.

b. Negatively impact dental health: Eating too much sugar can cause cavities. Bacteria in your mouth feed on sugar and release acid byproducts, which cause tooth demineralization.

c. Increase the risk of developing gout: Gout is an inflammatory condition characterized by pain in the joints. Added sugars raise uric acid levels in the blood, increasing the risk of developing or worsening gout.

d. Accelerate cognitive decline: High-sugar diets can lead to impaired memory and have been linked to an increased risk of dementia.

How to Reduce Your Sugar Intake:

1. You should drastically limit your consumption of sweets. Cookies, cakes, etc. These tend to be very high in sugar and refined carbohydrates. Instead of sugar in recipes, you can try things like cinnamon, nutmeg, almond extract, vanilla, ginger or lemon.

2. Swap sodas, energy drinks, juices and sweetened teas for water. Sugar-sweetened beverages are unhealthy. Drink water instead of soda or juices and don't add sugar to your tea.

3. Use Stevia in place of regular sugar

4. Sweeten plain yogurt with fresh or frozen berries instead of buying flavored, sugar-loaded yogurt.

5. Consume whole fruits instead of sugar-sweetened fruit smoothies. Fruit juices actually contain the same amount of sugar as soft drinks! Choose whole fruit instead of fruit juice. Avoid fruits canned in syrup.

6. Choose marinades, nut butters, ketchup and marinara sauce with zero added sugars.

7. Swap your morning cereal for a bowl of rolled oats topped with nut butter and fresh berries, or an omelet made with fresh greens.

8. Use natural nut butters in place of sweet.

9. Avoid alcoholic beverages that are sweetened with soda, juice, honey, sugar or agave.

10. Shop the perimeter of the grocery store, focusing on fresh, whole ingredients.

11.   Low-fat or diet foods that have had the fat removed from them are often
      very high in sugar.

In addition, keeping a food diary is an excellent way of becoming more aware
of the main sources of sugar in your diet. The best way to limit your added
sugar intake is to prepare your own healthy meals at home and avoid buying
foods and drinks that are high in added sugar.

A natural, zero-calorie alternative to sugar is stevia. Stevia plant is
a small, sweet, leafy herb. Stevia has no calories, and it is 200 times sweeter
than sugar in the same concentration. Other studies suggest stevia might have
extra health benefits.

Health benefits of stevia:

1.   Stevia herb parts are very low in calories. Parts by parts, its dry
     leaves possess roughly 40 times more sweetness than sugar. This sweetness
     quality in stevia is due to several glycoside compounds
     including stevioside, steviolbioside, rebaudiosides A-E, and dulcoside.

2.   Stevioside is a non-carbohydrate glycoside compound. Hence, it lacks the
     properties that sucrose and other carbohydrates possess. Stevia
     extracts, like rebaudioside-A, are found to be 300 times sweeter than
     sugar. Besides, being a near-zero calorie food ingredient, stevia
     extracts have several unique properties such as long shelf life, high-
     temperature tolerance, non-fermentative.

3.   Further, stevia plant has many sterols and antioxidant compounds
     like triterpenes, flavonoids, and tannins. Some of the flavonoid
     polyphenolic anti-oxidant phytochemicals present in stevia
     are kaempferol, quercetin, chlorogenic acid, caffeic acid,
     isoquercitrin, iso-steviol, etc. Studies found that kaempferol can
     reduce the risk of pancreatic cancer by 23% (American Journal of
     Epidemiology) [1].

4.   Chlorogenic acid in stevia reduces the enzymatic conversion of glycogen
     to glucose in addition to decreasing absorption of glucose in the gut.

Thus, it helps reduce blood sugar levels. Lab studies also confirm a reduction in blood glucose levels and an increase in the liver concentrations of glucose-6-phosphate, and of glycogen.

5. Certain glycosides in stevia extract have been found to dilate blood vessels, increase sodium excretion, and urine output. In effect, stevia, at slightly higher doses than as sweetener, can help lower blood pressure.

6. Being a non-carbohydrate sweetener, stevia would not favor the growth of Streptococcus mutans bacteria in the mouth which is attributed to be a causative agent of dental caries and tooth cavities. On the other hand, certain compounds in stevia rather found to inhibit caries-causing bacteria in the mouth.

7. Further, being an herb, stevia contains many vitals minerals, vitamins that are selectively absent in the artificial sweeteners.

Recently, the interest in attention-deficit hyperactivity disorder (ADHD) during childhood has increased. ADHD is defined as a neurobehavioral developmental disorder characterized by continuous inattention, hyperactivity, and impulsiveness and is especially prevalent in childhood. Unlike those showing simple hyperactivity features, children with ADHD have three subtype symptoms: predominantly hyperactive-impulsive, predominantly inattentive, and combined hyperactive-impulsive and inattentive.

Simple sugar consumption may cause hyperactivity, given that snacks containing high sugar content cause massive secretion of insulin from the pancreas, resulting in hypoglycemia. This stimulates an increase in epinephrine, leading to activation of nervous reactions and hyperactivity disorder behaviors. In other words, elevated intake of snacks might increase the potential of nutritional imbalance, lower emotional intelligence, and ADHD. A recent study on sugar consumption suggested that higher consumption of sugar is positively correlated with a higher level of hyperactivity and attention deficiency similar to ADHD. However, it is still controversial whether or not there is an association between ADHD and sugar consumption. A study found that diets high in sucrose had no significant effects on behavior and cognitive performance in children. Moreover, in Korea, there are little data on how much simple sugar children obtain from snacks or if higher consumption of simple sugar is associated with ADHD risk. Several recent studies suggested that ADHD development is related with consumption of coloring agents and preservatives in processed food.

Research undertaken by Southampton University appears to support Feingold's findings. It showed that consuming certain artificial food colors could impact a child's behavior. Thus, eliminating specific listed food colorings could improve behavior, especially in children with signs of hyperactivity or Attention Deficit Hyperactivity Disorder (ADHD). The study concludes that eliminating these colors could encourage positive behavioral changes. So, it seems there is a clear link between certain artificial additives and behavior.

Symptoms of inattention in children:

1. Has trouble staying focused; is easily distracted or gets bored with a task before it's completed

2. Appears not to listen when spoken to

3. Has difficulty remembering things and following instructions; doesn't pay attention to details or makes careless mistakes

4. Has trouble staying organized, planning ahead, and finishing projects

5. Frequently loses or misplaces homework, books, toys, or other items

The most obvious sign of ADHD is hyperactivity. While many children are naturally quite active, kids with hyperactive symptoms of attention deficit disorder are always moving. They may try to do several things at once, bouncing around from one activity to the next. Even when forced to sit still which can be very difficult for them their foot is tapping, their leg is shaking, or their fingers are drumming.

Symptoms of hyperactivity in children:

1. Constantly fidgets and squirms

2. Has difficulty sitting still, playing quietly, or relaxing

3. Moves around constantly, often runs or climbs inappropriately

4. Talks excessively

5. May have a quick temper or "short fuse"

The impulsivity of children with ADHD can cause problems with self-control. Because they censor themselves less than other kids do, they'll interrupt conversations, invade other people's space, ask irrelevant questions in class, make tactless observations, and ask overly personal questions. Instructions like "Be patient" and "Just wait a little while" are twice as hard for children with ADHD to follow as they are for other youngsters. Children with impulsive signs and symptoms of ADHD also tend to be moody and to overreact emotionally. As a result, others may start to view the child as disrespectful, weird, or needy.

Symptoms of impulsivity in children:

1. Acts without thinking

2. Guesses, rather than taking time to solve a problem or blurts out answers in class without waiting to be called on or hear the whole question

3. Intrudes on other people's conversations or games

4. Often interrupts others; says the wrong thing at the wrong time

5. Inability to keep powerful emotions in check, resulting in angry outbursts or temper tantrums

However, here's a list of additives that *could* aggravate attention problems, although none (with the exception of Yellow No. 5) has been studied alone in humans.

1. Blue No. 1 *also known as:* Brilliant blue

    Blue No. 2 *also known as:* Indigotine

    Green No. 3

2. Orange B

3. Red No. 3 *also known as:* Carmoisine

4. Sodium benzoate

5. Red No. 40 *also known as:* Allura red

6. Yellow No. 5 *also known as:* Tartrazine

7. Yellow No. 6 *also known as:* Sunset yellow

Several studies suggest that some kids who have ADHD are "turned on" by copious amounts of sugar. One study[5] concluded that the more sugar hyperactive children consumed, the more destructive and restless they became. A study conducted indicates that high-sugar diets increase inattention in some kids. Some common items to avoid include fruit "drinks" or "cocktails," both of which are higher in sugar than 100 percent fruit juice. Read food labels carefully, looking for the following ingredients (code words for sugar): high-fructose corn sweetener, dehydrated cane juice; dextrin; dextrose; maltodextrin; sucrose; molasses; and malt syrup. Studies published suggest that some children with ADHD are adversely affected by food additives. A recent study indicates that artificial food coloring and flavors, as well as the preservative sodium benzoate, make some kids without ADHD hyperactive. Avoid colorful cereals. According to studies, gluten, wheat, corn, and soy cause some children to lose focus and become more hyperactive. Experts suggest that all children be screened for food allergies before being prescribed medication for ADHD. Talk with your doctor about testing for allergies.

Deficiencies in certain types of foods can worsen symptoms of attention deficit disorder (ADHD or ADD) in children and adults. An ADHD diet that ensures you're getting adequate levels of the right foods optimizes brain function.

Recommended for ADHD:

1. Protein:

    Foods rich in protein — lean beef, pork, poultry, fish, eggs, beans, nuts, soy, and low-fat dairy products — can have beneficial effects on ADHD symptoms. Protein-rich foods are used by the body to make neurotransmitters, the chemicals released by brain cells to communicate with each other. Protein can prevent surges in blood sugar, which increase hyperactivity. Because the body makes brain-awakening neurotransmitters when you eat protein, start your day with a breakfast that includes it. Don't stop there. Look for ways to slip in lean protein during the day, as well.

2. Balanced Meals:

    Medication for ADHD may not be enough. Eating a well-balanced diet, including vegetables, complex carbohydrates, fruits, and plenty of protein, may result in behavior consistently under control.

3. Zinc, Iron, and Magnesium:

    Zinc regulates the neurotransmitter dopamine and may make methylphenidate more effective by improving the brain's response to dopamine. Low levels of this mineral correlate with inattention. Iron is also necessary for making dopamine. One small study showed ferritin levels (a measure of iron stores) to be low in 84 percent of children with ADHD compared to 18 percent of the control group. Low iron levels correlate with cognitive deficits and severe ADHD. Like zinc, magnesium is used to make neurotransmitters involved in attention and concentration, and it has a calming effect on the brain. All three minerals are found in lean meats, poultry, seafood, nuts, and soy. While diet is the safest way to increase all three mineral levels, a multivitamin/multimineral with iron will ensure that you or your child gets the daily reference value (DRV) of these minerals. Many diets are deficient in key vitamins, minerals, and fats that may improve attention and alertness. Experts suggest having children and adults who have been diagnosed with ADHD be tested for nutritional deficiencies. Supplements and diet can correct nutrient shortfalls that exacerbate ADHD symptoms.

4.   B Vitamins:

Studies suggest that giving children who have low levels of B vitamins a supplement improved some IQ scores (by 16 points) and reduced aggression and antisocial behavior. Vitamin B-6 seems to increase the brain's levels of dopamine, which improves alertness.

5.   Multivitamin/Multimineral:

If your child is a picky eater, or if he eats lots of take-out food, chips, and soda, he probably isn't getting the daily recommended value of vitamins and minerals. A daily multivitamin/multimineral will ensure that he does, no matter how finicky the child is. Children diagnosed with ADHD should take multi-vitamins or multi-minerals that does not contain artificial colors and flavors, which increase hyperactivity in some children with ADHD.

6.   Picamilon:

A combination of the B-vitamin niacin and gamma-aminobutyric acid (GABA), picamilon improves blood flow to the brain and has mild simulative effects, improving alertness and attention. It can also reduce aggressive behavior. Both adults and children derive benefits from this supplement.

7.   Omega-3 Fatty Acids:

Omega-3s are believed to be important in brain and nerve cell function. A new study concluded that daily doses of omega-3s — found in cold-water, fatty fish, such as sardines, tuna, and salmon — reduced ADHD symptoms by 50 percent. A study was conducted on a group of ADHD children aged 8-18 who took fish oil daily. Within six months, there was a noticeable decrease in ADHD symptoms in 25 percent of the children. Another study showed that omega-3s tend to break down more readily in the bodies of patients with ADHD than in those without the condition. People with ADHD who have low blood levels of omega-3s will show the biggest improvement in mental focus and cognitive function. Sometimes the change is dramatic. Experts recommends a supplement that contains more EPA (eicosapentaenoic acid) than DHA (docosahexaenoic acid).

Herbs may improve blood flow to the brain, increasing alertness while reducing aggressive behavior. Talk with your doctor, or a psycho-pharmacologist, before starting an herb regimen.

1. Ginkgo and Ginseng:

These herbs are cognitive activators. They act like stimulants, without the side effects of ADHD medication. Typically, adults and children who take ginkgo and ginseng improve on ADHD rating scales and are less impulsive and distractible. Asian ginseng may overstimulate younger children. If this happens, switch to American ginseng.

2. Pycnogenol:

Pycnogenol was found to improve hyperactivity and sharpen attention, concentration, and visual-motor coordination in students after one month, based on standardized measures and teacher and parent ratings. The herb is also rich in polyphenols, antioxidants that protect brain cells from free radical damage.

3. Rhodiola Rosea:

This herb can improve alertness, attention, and accuracy. It can be too stimulating for young children and is occasionally beneficial in children ages eight to 12. It is most useful for students in junior high, high school, and college, who have to complete long papers and spend hours reading.

Speaking of sugar, I could not leave coffee out of this discussion. I made the decision not cut caffeine completely out of my life. Some experts believe there are benefits of consuming coffee in moderation while others believe coffee offers no benefits.

Coffee may raise cholesterol, but this depends on how you brew it and how much you drink. If you're sensitive to caffeine, coffee may also impact your health. Several studies over the past decade have shown a link between coffee and cholesterol. According to one study, coffee oils (known as diterpenes) such as cafestol and kahweol are to blame. Coffee oils are naturally found in caffeinated and decaffeinated coffee. Research indicates that cafestol affects the body's ability to metabolize and regulate cholesterol. According to a meta-analysis of controlled studies on coffee and cholesterol, coffee oils may decrease bile acids and neutral sterols. This may lead to increased cholesterol. Researchers concluded that cafestol is the "most potent cholesterol-elevating compound identified in the human diet. If you have a genetic mutation that slows down coffee metabolism in your body, and you drink two or more cups of coffee a day, your risk of heart disease may be higher.

Coffee oils are most potent in coffees where the grounds have the longest contact with the water during brewing. A French press, which brews coffee by continually passing water through the grounds, has been shown to have greater concentrations of cafestol. Brewing in an American-style coffee pot with a filter, on the other hand, has relatively low levels, as the beverage is only passed through the grounds once. Most of the cafestol is left behind in the filter no matter what the roast. Another study found that Turkish-style simmered coffee and Scandinavian-style boiled coffee had the highest amount of diterpenes. Instant coffee and drip-brewed coffee had "negligible" amounts, and espresso had intermediate amounts. Research has shown that drinking five cups of coffee daily from a French press brewing method can increase blood cholesterol levels by 6 to 8 percent.

Up to four hundred milligrams (mg) of caffeine a day appears to be safe for most healthy adults. That's roughly the amount of caffeine in four cups of brewed coffee, 10 cans of cola or two "energy shot" drinks. Keep in mind that the actual caffeine content in beverages varies widely, especially among energy drinks. Although caffeine use may be safe for adults, it's not a good idea for children. Adolescents should limit caffeine consumption. Avoid mixing caffeine with other substances, such as alcohol. Even among adults, heavy caffeine use can cause unpleasant side effects. And caffeine may not be a good choice for people who are highly sensitive to its effects or who take certain medications. Women who are pregnant or who are trying to become pregnant and those who are breastfeeding should talk with their doctors about limiting caffeine use. Read on to see if you may need to curb your caffeine routine.

You may want to cut back if you're drinking more than 4 cups of caffeinated coffee a day (or the equivalent) and you're experiencing side effects such as:

1. Migraine headache
2. Insomnia

3.   Nervousness

4.   Irritability

5.   Restlessness

6.   Frequent urination or inability to control urination

7.   Stomach upset

8.   Fast heartbeat

9.   Muscle tremors

Some people are more sensitive to caffeine than are others. Even a little makes some jittery. If you're susceptible to the effects of caffeine, just small amounts — even one cup of coffee or tea — may prompt unwanted effects, such as restlessness and sleep problems. How you react to caffeine may be determined in part by how much caffeine you're used to drinking. People who don't regularly drink caffeine tend to be more sensitive to its negative effects. Other factors may include genetics, body mass, age, medication use and health conditions, such as anxiety disorders.

Most adults need seven to eight hours of sleep each night. But caffeine, even in the afternoon, can interfere with this much-needed sleep. Chronically losing sleep — whether it's from work, travel, stress or too much caffeine — results in sleep deprivation. Sleep loss is cumulative, and even small nightly decreases can add up and disturb your daytime alertness and performance. Using caffeine to mask sleep deprivation can create an unwelcome cycle. For example, you may drink caffeinated beverages because you have trouble staying awake during the day. But the caffeine keeps you from falling asleep at night, shortening the length of time you sleep.

Certain medications and herbal supplements may interact with caffeine.

Examples include:

1.   Ephedrine: Mixing caffeine with this medication — which is used in decongestants — might increase your risk of high blood pressure, heart attack, stroke or seizure.

2.   Theophylline (Theo-24, Elixophyllin, others): This medication, used to open up bronchial airways, tends to have some caffeine-like effects. So,

taking it with caffeine might increase the adverse effects of caffeine, such as nausea and heart palpitations.

3. Echinacea: This herbal supplement, which is sometimes used to prevent colds or other infections, may increase the concentration of caffeine in your blood and may increase caffeine's unpleasant effects.

Talk to your doctor or pharmacist about whether caffeine might affect your medications.

Whether it's for one of the reasons above — or because you want to trim your spending on coffee drinks — cutting back on caffeine can be challenging. An abrupt decrease in caffeine may cause withdrawal symptoms, such as headaches, fatigue, irritability and difficulty focusing on tasks. Fortunately, these symptoms are usually mild and resolve after a few days.

To change your caffeine habit, try these tips:

1. Keep tabs: Start paying attention to how much caffeine you're getting from foods and beverages, including energy drinks. Read labels carefully. But remember that your estimate may be a little low because some foods or drinks that contain caffeine don't list it.

2. Cut back gradually: For example, drink one fewer can of soda or drink a smaller cup of coffee each day. Or avoid drinking caffeinated beverages late in the day. This will help your body get used to the lower levels of caffeine and lessen potential withdrawal effects.

3. Go decaf: Most decaffeinated beverages look and taste the same as their caffeinated counterparts.

4. Shorten the brew time or go herbal: When making tea, brew it for less time. This cuts down on its caffeine content. Or choose herbal teas that don't have caffeine.

5. Check the bottle: Some over-the-counter pain relievers contain caffeine — as much as 130 mg of caffeine in one dose. Look for caffeine-free pain relievers instead.

Reasons to quit coffee:

1. The caffeine in coffee increases catecholamines, your stress hormones. The stress response elicits cortisol and increases insulin. Insulin increases inflammation.

2. Habituation to caffeine decreases insulin sensitivity, making it difficult for your cells to respond appropriately to blood sugar. High blood sugar levels lead to arterial deterioration and increased risk of mortality related cardiovascular disease.

3. Unfiltered coffee has the highest number of beneficial antioxidants yet also leaks the most diterpenes into your system. These diterpenes have been linked to higher levels of triglycerides, LDL and VLDL levels. The helpful chlorogenic acids that may delay glucose absorption in the intestine have also been shown to increase homocysteine levels – an indicator for increased risk of cardiovascular disease, which tends to be elevated in diabesity.

4. The acidity of coffee is associated with digestive discomfort, indigestion, heart burn, GERD, and dysbiosis (imbalances in gut flora).

5. Addiction is often an issue with coffee drinkers and makes it really difficult to rely on the body's natural source of energy. If you were to ask any coffee drinker about how it feels to withdraw from coffee, you can easily mistake their story for someone struggling with an addiction.

6. HIA, an organic acid and component of the neurotransmitter serotonin (the happy chemical) seen in urine tends to be elevated in coffee drinkers, which means they may be at risk for lower levels of serotonin synthesis in the brain. Serotonin is necessary for normal sleep, bowel function, mood, and energy levels. Caffeine can disrupt sleep, and promote anxiety, and promote depression. This is especially true when you think of some people who are tired, wired, and over-caffeinated.

7. Elevated urinary excretion of important minerals such as calcium, magnesium, and potassium have been noted in coffee drinkers. An imbalance in electrolyte status can lead to serious complications.

8. Constituents in coffee can interfere with normal drug metabolism and detoxification in the liver, making it difficult to regulate the normal

detoxification process in the liver, another issue to be aware of with coffee intake is how certain medications and tricyclic antidepressants are poorly absorbed, making symptoms curiously worse for patients.

Withdrawal symptoms tend to disappear after three or four days. However, the length of time a person experiences withdrawal symptom may or may not be impacted the volume of coffee and length of time this person consumed coffee.

How to avoid withdrawal symptoms:

1.   Make sure you drink at least six to eight glasses of filtered water daily instead of drinking coffee. You can even squeeze a lemon over your water and add stevia.
2.   The best water to drink is water that has been passed through a filtering process. The best filter is a reverse osmosis filter that puts the water through a multi-step process to remove microbes, pesticides, metals, and other toxins. This filter can be installed underneath your sink.
3.   Avoid water in plastic bottles, which contains phthalates, a toxic petrochemical. Mineral water or still water in glass bottles is also acceptable.
4.   To prevent headaches, make sure your bowel movements are regular.
5.   If you are tired, allow more time for sleep.
6.   Take 1,000 mg (milligrams) buffered vitamin C with breakfast and dinner. You might also want to consider taking a good multi-vitamin.
7.   Make sure you exercise daily to help fight off fatigue.
8.   Substitute coffee for real food. Eat when you are hungry to avoid low blood sugar. Have some protein in the afternoon.
9.   If you are experiencing irritability or have trouble sleeping, take a combination of calcium 500 mg (milligrams) and magnesium 250 mg (milligrams) before bed time.
10.   Take a sauna or heat therapy in a bath.
11.   Make a decision not to be stressed.
12.   Keep a journal. Track any withdrawal symptoms. Note the difference in quality of energy you have without drinking coffee.
13.   Consider a complete elimination program. Avoid all refined sugars, flours, caffeine, alcohol, diary, gluten, and any other addictive

substance. Reset your biology by eliminating all these dietary triggers for inflammation and fatigue.

Energy drinks, shots, and other energy products contain large amounts of caffeine, and an assortment of other ingredients. Heavy consumption of energy drinks may result in excessive consumption of B vitamins, such as niacin or pyridoxine, and may result in liver or nerve injury. Alcohol mixed with caffeinated energy drinks puts adolescents and young adults at serious risk of self-harm and other harm.

Medical researchers have more to learn about energy drinks, but the primary cause of serious health problems appears to be the high concentrations of caffeine.

Examples of findings related to cardiovascular effects are:

1. Heart palpitations: According to one study, 19 percent of college students who used energy drinks had experienced heart palpitations.

2. Increased heart rate and blood pressure: Energy drinks can increase heart rate and blood pressure, particularly in people who already have heart disease.

The risks associated with energy drinks are believed to be higher for people who have existing medical conditions, such as heart defects or certain heart conditions. For example, people with hypertrophic cardiomyopathy should not have caffeine or other stimulants, as they may increase the risk of irregular heart rhythms, high blood pressure, and sudden death from cardiac arrest.

15 Possible Dangers of Consuming Energy Drinks:

1. Cardiac Arrest: Although a Caffeine Calculator can show people how many energy drinks at one time would be lethal, this formula doesn't apply to everyone. Those with underlying heart conditions have gone into cardiac arrest after just a few energy drinks. Before drinking energy drinks or caffeine, be sure to know your heart's health. A new study showed that energy drinks cause more forceful heart contractions, which could be

harmful to some with certain heart conditions. A 2016 study showed that 18-40-year-olds who drank energy drinks had a significant increase in their QTc interval, which is a marker of abnormal heart rhythm risk. Research in 2018 showed that just 90 minutes after consuming a 24-oz energy drink, the inner diameter of arteries was halved. It's thought that the high level of sugar and caffeine were to blame.

2. Headaches and Migraines: Too many energy drinks can lead to severe headaches from the caffeine withdrawal symptoms. Changing the amount of caffeine, you ingest daily can cause more frequent headaches.

3. Increased Anxiety: Those with 2 different genetic variations in their adenosine receptors are prone to feeling increased anxiety when consuming caffeinated beverages such as energy drinks. Larger doses of caffeine can even spur on full-blown panic attacks.

4. Insomnia: Energy drinks do a good job of keeping people awake, but when abused, they can cause some people to miss sleep altogether. This lack of sleep causes impaired functioning and can be dangerous to drive or perform other concentration heavy tasks.

5. Type 2 Diabetes: Because many energy drinks are also very high in sugar, they can eventually wear out the insulin-producing cells of the pancreas, which leads to type 2 diabetes. High consumption of caffeine reduces insulin sensitivity.

6. Drug Interaction: Some of the ingredients in energy drinks can interact with prescription medications especially medications taken for depression.

7. Addiction: People can become addicted to caffeine and energy drinks. This can lead to a lack of functioning when unable to have the energy drink or a financial stress from having to buy several energy drinks daily. This may also lead to use and dependence on other harmful substances.

8. Risky behavior: There was a study published in The Journal of American College Health which showed that teens are more likely to take dangerous

risks or engage in sensation seeking behavior when high on caffeine. This could result in injury or legal trouble.

9. Jitters and Nervousness: Too much caffeine from energy drinks causes some people to shake and be anxious. This can interfere with performing needed tasks or cause emotional issues. This study shows how caffeine can elicit anxiety.

10. Vomiting: Too many energy drinks can lead to vomiting. This causes dehydration and acid erosion of teeth and esophagus if frequent.

11. Allergic Reactions: Because of the many ingredients in energy drinks reactions could occur, from minor itching to airway constriction.

12. High Blood Pressure: Caffeinated products like energy drinks can elevate a person's blood pressure. For those with normal blood pressure, this isn't concerning, but those with already elevated blood pressure could be placing themselves at risk of stroke and other health problems related to hypertension if they consume too many energy drinks in a short period of time. A more recent study conducted by The Mayo Clinic found that Rockstar Energy Drink (240 mg version) significantly raised the blood pressure of study participants compared to the placebo drink. Overall, there was a 6.4% increase in average blood pressure. A newer study published by the American Heart Associations showed that energy drinks have a greater negative effect on blood pressure than drinks that contain caffeine alone as the active ingredient. They believe the combination of ingredients in energy drinks are why these beverages pose a greater risk of heart-related problems than drinks like coffee or tea.

13. Niacin Overdose: Niacin (Vitamin B3) is placed in most energy drinks at levels that cause no harm and can even be therapeutic. However, if a person is taking additional supplements containing Niacin, overdosing on the vitamin is possible when consuming energy drinks in addition to those supplements. Symptoms include; Skin flushing, dizziness, rapid heart rate, vomiting, itching, gout, and diarrhea. The British Journal of Medicine recently published a case study of a man who experienced nonviral

hepatitis from B3 toxicity believed to have been from consuming too many energy drinks during a period of three weeks.

14. Stress Hormone Release: A study conducted by The Mayo Clinic found that a 240 mg version of Rockstar Energy Drink caused an increase in stress hormone release. The average norepinephrine level of the participants increased by 74% while the placebo only caused a 31% increase.

15. Mental Health Problems, Aggression, and Fatigue. A recent study conducted by the US Military found that soldiers who drink 2+ energy drinks a day are more likely to exhibit mental health issues, aggression, and fatigue. Neurological and cardiovascular system effects in children and adolescents.

16. Caffeine overdose (which can lead to a number of symptoms, including palpitations, high blood pressure, nausea, and vomiting, convulsions, and in some cases even death)

17. Late miscarriages, low birthweight, and stillbirths in pregnant women

18. Poor dental health

Both vegetarians and vegans have to be sure the complete spectrum of their nutritional needs are met. This means eating a <u>balanced selection of foods</u> to get their daily nutritional requirements of zinc, iron, calcium, and protein. Having a very diverse diet and taking advantage of all the food choices available is a great step in the right direction to getting all the nutrients your body needs. Popular foods among both vegetarians and vegans include kale, nuts, legumes, and beans. Because processed foods are avoided, having vegan diet habits is a great way to get into the kitchen and prepare your own healthy and delicious dishes!

Vegans who take nutritional supplements have to be especially aware that just because nutritional supplements are marketed as "natural and healthy" doesn't automatically mean they're truly vegan safe (or even beneficial at all). When investing in vitamins or body cleansing products, make sure you only do business with a reputable company that stands by their products and divulges where and how things were produced. Avoid the slick ads that promise everything and explain nothing. Quality is not an appropriate category to cut corners.

Vegans tend to have a vitamin B12 deficiency. Vitamin B12 is only found in substantial amounts through animal foods. For this reason, several studies have found that vegans and vegetarians have a higher tendency and risk to be B12 deficient. Vitamin B12 is essential for energy metabolism in cells, proper brain function, red blood cell formation, among many other body processes. B12 deficiency can cause anemia, depression, fatigue, and much more. To support the body and overall health, supplement your diet with a quality B12 product. It important not only for vegans and vegetarians but omnivores, too.

Some people believe meat has little to no nutritional value. Chicken has some nutritional value. Despite popular belief, red meat can be very nutritious. Red meat is loaded with vitamins, minerals, antioxidants and various other nutrients that can have profound effects on health. The nutritional value of red meat is largely determined by how it is prepared. Red meat is also rich in important nutrients like creatine and carnosine. Non-meat eaters are often low in these nutrients, which may potentially affect muscle and brain function.

A 3.5-ounce (100-gram) portion of raw ground beef (10% fat) contains:

1. Vitamin B3 (niacin): 25% of the RDA

2. Vitamin B12 (cobalamin): 37% of the RDA (this vitamin is unattainable from plant foods)

3. Vitamin B6 (pyridoxine): 18% of the RDA

4. Iron: 12% of the RDA (this is high-quality heme iron, which is absorbed much better than iron from plants)

5. Zinc: 32% of the RDA

6. Selenium: 24% of the RDA

7.   Plenty of other vitamins and minerals in smaller amounts

This comes with a calorie count of 176, with 20 grams of quality animal protein and 10 grams of fat.

People who like their steak well-done instead of rare might face a slightly increased risk of high blood pressure, a preliminary study suggests. Research suggests that cooking to the point of "charring" is the main issue. The process produces chemicals that are not normally present in the body. These chemicals include heterocyclic amines (HAs), polycyclic aromatic hydrocarbons (PAHs) and advanced glycation end-products (AGEs). Studies suggest these chemicals can trigger inflammation within the body, which could contribute to high blood pressure and other health problems. Meanwhile, studies have found that people who eat a lot of well-done meat tend to face increased risks of certain cancers, as well as heart disease and type 2 diabetes.

Here are some tips to ensure your meat doesn't form these harmful substances:

1. Use gentler cooking methods like baking, stewing, and steaming instead of grilling and frying.

2. Minimize cooking at high heats and never expose your meat to a flame.

3. Do not eat charred and/or smoked food. If your meat is burnt, cut away the charred pieces.

4. If you marinate your meat in garlic, red wine, or lemon juice, it can reduce HAs significantly.

5. If you must cook at a high heat, flip your meat frequently to prevent it from burning.

Many people love the taste of fried and grilled meat. But if you want to enjoy meat and receive the full benefits without any of the potentially harmful consequences, use gentler cooking methods and avoid burnt meat.

I don't know whether or not you have heard of nitrates in processed meats such as salami, bologna, bacon, etc. Nitrates and Nitrites are compounds consisting of Nitrogen and Oxygen atoms. Nitrates can turn into Nitrites, which can then form either Nitric Oxide (good) or Nitrosamines (bad). Nitrates are found in small amounts in processed meats, and in much larger amounts in healthy foods like vegetables. They are also found in drinking water and produced in our own bodies.

Nitrates and nitrites are frequently added to processed meats like bacon, ham, sausages and hot dogs. Our bodies also produce nitrates in large amounts and secrete them into saliva. Nitrates and nitrites actually circulate from the digestive system, into the blood, then into saliva and then back into the digestive system. This is known as the entero-salivary circulation. They seem to function as antimicrobials in the digestive system, helping to kill pathogenic bacteria like Salmonella. They can also turn into Nitric Oxide (NO), an important signaling molecule.

Nitrates can even be found in drinking water in some areas. This can be a problem for infants under 6 months of age, which are unable to process a lot of nitrate. This can lead to a dangerous condition called methemoglobinemia, which is why nitrate amounts in drinking water are regulated. However, this is not a problem in adults or older children, who can process nitrates just fine.

If nitrite loses an oxygen atom, it turns into Nitric Oxide, an important molecule. Nitric Oxide (NO) is a short-lived gas, which has various functions in the body. Most importantly, it is a signaling molecule. It travels through the artery wall and sends signals to the tiny muscle cells around the arteries, telling them to relax. When these cells relax, our blood vessels dilate and blood pressure goes down. This is actually how the well-known drug nitroglycerin works. It is a source of nitrate, which quickly turns into nitric oxide and dilates the blood vessels. This can prevent or reverse angina, chest pain that occurs when the heart muscle doesn't get enough oxygen due to reduced blood flow. Dietary nitrates and nitrites can also turn into Nitric Oxide, dilate the blood vessels and lower blood pressure.

There is a lot of confusion about Nitrates and Nitrites in the diet. These are compounds found naturally in some foods (like vegetables) but also added to processed foods (like bacon) as a preservative. Some people believe that they are harmful and can cause cancer. However, the science isn't as clear and some studies suggest that they may even be healthy.

These are two types of compounds, consisting of a single Nitrogen atom bonded to a number of Oxygen atoms:

1.   Nitrate: 1 Nitrogen, 3 Oxygens - Chemical Formula: NO3-

2.   Nitrite: 1 Nitrogen, 2 Oxygens - Chemical Formula: NO2-

So... Nitr-a-tes have 3 oxygen atoms, while Nitr-i-tes have 2 oxygen atoms.

This is what they look like:

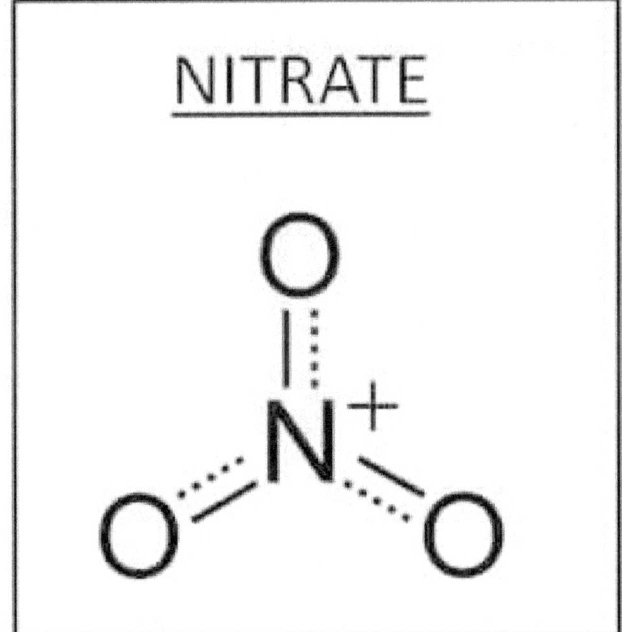

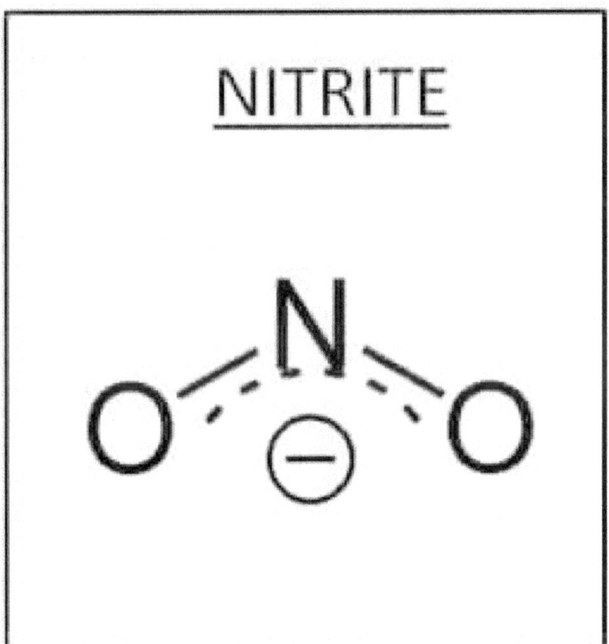

It seems that the nitrates themselves are relatively inert, until they are turned into nitrites by bacteria in the mouth or enzymes in the body. Nitrites are the key players here... they can either turn into Nitric Oxide (good) or nitrosamines (bad). Nitrites are the reason cured meat is pink or red. Nitrites turn into Nitric Oxide, which reacts with the oxygen-binding proteins in the meat, changing its color. Without additives like nitrites, the meat would turn brown very quickly. We do know that consuming processed meats is strongly linked to an increased risk of cancer in the digestive tract, and many people believe that the nitrates/nitrites are the reason for that.

However, they are also found naturally in foods like vegetables, foods that are generally perceived as healthy and linked to a reduced risk of cancer. Vegetables are actually the biggest dietary source of nitrates... by far. The amount you get from processed meat is small compared to vegetables.

Our bodies also produce nitrates in large amounts and secrete them into saliva. Nitrates and nitrites actually circulate from the digestive system, into the blood, then into saliva and then back into the digestive system. This is known as the entero-salivary circulation. They seem to function as antimicrobials in the digestive system, helping to kill pathogenic bacteria like Salmonella. They can also turn into Nitric Oxide (NO), an important signaling molecule.

Some experts believe nitrites are only a problem when they form nitrosamines. When nitrites are exposed to high heat, in the presence of amino acids, they can turn into compounds called nitrosamines. There are many different types of nitrosamines and most of them are potent carcinogens. They are among the main carcinogens in tobacco smoke, for example. Because most bacon, hot dogs and processed meat tend to be high in sodium nitrite *and* they're high protein foods (a source of amino acids), exposing them to high heat creates the perfect conditions for nitrosamine formation. It's important to keep in mind that nitrosamines mostly form during very high heat. Even though vegetables also contain nitrates/nitrites, they are rarely exposed to such high heat. Nitrosamines can also form during the acidic conditions in the stomach.

Nitrosamines are a well-known problem in processed meats, and manufacturers are required to limit the number of nitrites they use. They are also required to add Vitamin C, which inhibits nitrosamine formation. The processed meat eaten today contains about 80% less nitrites than it did a few decades ago. For these reasons, today's processed meat may not be nearly as carcinogenic as it used to be.

Uncured meat products are those that do not contain nitrate or nitrite. Within this category, you can find meat products in stores with the word "uncured" printed on the product label. This describes products traditionally required or expected to contain curing ingredients but allowed to be made without nitrate and nitrite as long as the word "uncured" is added to the package label. Natural meat products are those manufactured under stricter rules than traditional products which require minimal processing and also do not allow any added artificial coloring, flavoring, or preservatives. Because nitrate and nitrite used for traditional products are made by purification, they are not allowed. Organic meat products must follow standards established by the National Organic Program and governed by the USDA Organic Foods Production Act regarding practices and substances that may be used for production, processing, and handling of organic foods. Both purified nitrate and nitrite are listed as prohibited ingredients and as such may not be used.

Modern production of foods incorporates a wide range of synthetic chemicals. There are pesticides in produce, hormones in milk, and antibiotics and steroids in meat. Many of these chemicals have the potential to be very damaging to humans if they are exposed to high concentrations, or to low concentrations over an extended period of time. More people are realizing there's a myriad of chemicals in conventionally produced food.

Most beef cattle entering feedlots in the United States are given hormone implants to promote faster growth. The first product used for this purpose DES (diethylstilbestrol) was approved for use in beef cattle in 1954. Initial concerns about estrogen-injected cows centered on a compound called diethylstilbestrol (DES). Nearly all beef cattle were treated with DES in the 1950s and 1960s. DES was also used as medicine, given to pregnant women to prevent miscarriages. However, it was also discovered that DES caused a higher risk of vaginal cancer in the daughters of women who received the medicine. By the 1970s, over the protests of ranchers, diethylstilbestrol was phased out from use in medicine and agriculture.

Today are six anabolic steroids given, in various combinations, to nearly all animals entering conventional beef feedlots in the U.S. and Canada:

1.   Three natural steroids (estradiol, testosterone, and progesterone)
2.   Three synthetic hormones (the estrogen compound zeranol, the androgen trenbolone acetate, and progestin melengestrol acetate).

Anabolic steroids are typically used in combinations. Measurable levels of all the above growth-promoting hormones are found at slaughter in the muscle, fat, liver, kidneys and other organ meats. The Food and Drug Administration has set "acceptable daily intakes" (ADIs) for these animal drugs.

Injecting hormones into young livestock can make them gain weight faster. More weight means more meat, which means more profit for the producer. Hormones also increase the production of milk by dairy cows. Hormones have been used for decades in the meat and dairy industries. Synthetic estrogens and testosterone are the most common. Typically, farmers implant a pellet in a cow's ear at an early age; it releases hormones throughout the animal's life. It's also long been known that breast cancer risk increases with higher lifetime exposure to estrogen. These facts have led many to question whether the continued use of synthetic estrogens in livestock is safe.

Recombinant bovine growth hormone (rBGH) is a different class of hormone that increases the amount of milk dairy cows produce. Some suggest that although rBGH itself appears safe, it increases the amount of other chemicals in the body that might cause cancer. Responding to the lack of certainty, the European Union has banned all hormones in beef, and Japan, Canada, Australia, New Zealand, and the EU have banned rBGH. No major studies are under way in the U.S. to evaluate the safety of hormones in meat and milk.

The concern with conventional beef is the risk that cows may be given growth hormones (BGH, rBGH, rBST) to increase milk production in dairy cows or speed up and increase the size of cows that will go to slaughter for beef. Studies are inconclusive about how much humans can absorb the byproducts of these hormones, which have been linked to certain cancers, but a surefire way to avoid them is by eating organically raised cows, which are never given endogenous growth hormones. Antibiotics are prevalent in conventional chickens and can be preserved in the chicken we eat at the dinner table. Limiting sources of antibiotics is important because <u>antibiotic resistance</u> is a real problem.

Hormone-treated meat has long been suspected of contributing to early puberty in children, although the link has not been proven. There's no question that the age of puberty has been decreasing in the U.S. But some suggest that's due to improved nutrition and health, not to second helpings of hormones in children's diets. The effects are very hard to study, experts say, because hormones are naturally present in both food and our bodies. Plus, the effects could be subtle and take years to show up. The amount of hormone that enters a person's bloodstream after eating hormone-treated meat is small compared with the amount of estrogen a person produces daily. However, even low levels of hormones can have strong effects on some body processes.

There is a rampant use of antibiotics with livestock, which is primarily used as a tool to help them grow larger and bigger. Seventy percent of all antibiotics used in the U.S. is for livestock use. antibiotics aren't the only drugs given to livestock to help them grow faster. Each year, U.S. farmers raise some 36 million beef cattle. 99% of all beef cattle entering feedlots in the United States are given steroidal hormone implants to promote faster growth. A large percentage of poultry and pigs are also fed these drugs. Many cattle are fed the same muscle-building androgens—usually testosterone surrogates—that some athletes consume. Other animals receive estrogens, the primary female sex hormones, or progestins, semi androgenic agents that shut down a female's estrus cycle. Progestins fuel meat-building by freeing up resources that would have gone into the reproductive cycle.

Flunix is a steroidal hormone fed to livestock. While federal law prohibits people from self-medicating with most steroids, administering these drugs to U.S. cattle is allowed.

So, this means that when you eat meat, chicken or pork injected with antibiotics and steroids, and drink milk, you are consuming unsafe drugs that weren't prescribed to you. Consuming extra hormones disturbs the natural hormonal balance in the body and eating animal products laced with hormones can have serious consequences for both children and adults. Kids' bodies are small and still developing, so exposure to even tiny amounts of the hormones in animal products on a regular basis can have a large impact. The amount of estradiol in two hamburgers eaten in one day by an 8-year-old could increase his total hormone levels by as much as 10 percent, based on conservative assumptions, because young children have very low natural hormone levels.

The Cancer Prevention Coalition warns parents that even small amounts of animal products contain enough hormonal residues to harm children. No dietary levels of hormones are safe, and a dime-sized piece of meat contains billions of hormone molecules. When kids eat the flesh of cows who were treated with hormones, the spike in hormone levels can disrupt the development of their brain and sex organs. Certain organs are more susceptible to the effects of estrogens, androgens, and anti-androgens [all hormones used in cows raised for food] during development than during adulthood. These organs include the brain, and the primary and secondary sex organs.

The negative consequences of feeding children meat were clearly demonstrated in the early 1980s, when thousands of children experienced premature sexual development and painful ovarian cysts; the culprit was meat from cattle who had been treated with growth-promoting sex hormones.

Rimadyl is another steroid fed to livestock. The hormones in meat-based diets are also blamed for the early sexual development of young girls in the Western world. Rimadyl is responsible for some girls entering into puberty as early as 8 years old.

Raising the amount of estrogen and other hormones in our bodies through the consumption of meat and milk can cause other disorders, including gynecomastia, or enlarged male breasts. In one school in Italy, nearly one in three boys aged 3 to 5 and more than half of boys aged 6 to 10 were found to have enlarged breasts, and the hormones in meat were suspected to have caused the disorder. And that's just the known effects it has on children. For adults, it can have all kinds of repercussions, from hormonal imbalances, to auto-immune problems, cancer, liver and kidney failure, and all kinds of other things.

This is the type of meat you want to eat - antibiotic and hormone free. Some accuse the U.S. FDA of not adequately regulating the use of antibiotics and steroids to promote growth in cows, even though these very same drugs in the U.S. are prohibited for over-the-counter use by humans.

Studies have shown that <u>buying organic fruits and vegetables</u> to avoid ingesting dangerous chemicals and perhaps gaining more nutritional value from your produce is sometimes worthwhile. The same may be true to organic meats.

The United States Department of Agriculture <u>National Organic Program</u> defines organic food in the following way:

Organic food is produced by farmers who emphasize the use of renewable resources and the conservation of soil and water to enhance environmental quality for future generations. Organic meat, poultry, eggs and dairy products come from animals that are given no antibiotics or growth hormones. Organic food is produced without using most conventional pesticides; fertilizers made with synthetic ingredients or sewage sludge; bioengineering; or ionizing radiation. Before a product can be labeled "organic," a government-approved certifier inspects the farm where the food is grown to make sure the farmer is following all the rules necessary to meet USDA organic standards. Companies that handle or process organic food before it gets to your local supermarket or restaurant must be certified, too.

For an animal to be considered organic, the <u>USDA regulates several standards</u>. Beyond eating organic feed and being free of hormone injections, an organic animal must spend time outdoors and have enough space to live what the USDA defines as comfortably. Free range refers to food from animals, for example, meat or eggs, that are produced from animals that have access to outdoor spaces. Usually, free range also stands for animals who have free access to graze or forage for food. The USDA's <u>organic standards for</u>

livestock stipulate that cattle must be able to graze in an organic pasture for at least 120 days during grazing season. That four months of the year, however, is just a sliver of a cattle's lifespan: Most beef cattle are slaughtered at about 18-22 months of age, meaning that most of your grass-fed organic beef's life may have been spent eating organic feed (like hay and alfalfa pellets) rather than grass. Organic grass-fed meat comes from animals that have been naturally fed and raised organically, without drugs and hormones. They also don't have any artificial chemicals added. Grass-fed beef is even more nutritious than grain-fed beef, containing plenty of heart-healthy omega-3s, the fatty acid CLA and higher amounts of vitamins A and E. If you're committed to eating 100% grass-fed beef, either because you prefer the taste, are health conscious (cattle fed a mostly-grass diet have higher levels of omega-3s, more antioxidants, can have lower levels of fat and are considered more nutritious) or are just looking for a steak to comply with your paleo diet, you should look for a trusted third-party verification on the package, like the American Grass-fed approved logo. If that's a no-go, search for the phrase "grass-finished".

The USDA strictly specifies what products can be labeled organic or not. Not all organic meat, however, is labeled as such. Getting organic certification is expensive and for farmers operating small farms, the certification may not be worthwhile. Not using antibiotics can also be expensive for small farmers, who may rather help an animal recover from disease or sickness than let them die because they cannot use antibiotics to heal their livestock. Small farmers and conventional farmers who are not organic may also choose to abstain from using hormones and steroids which quicken the growth of livestock. Hormones given to poultry and livestock correlate to a higher rate of hormone-dependent cancers, which is why some prefer to eat hormone-free meats, though those are not necessarily organic.

Pork is the most widely eaten meat in the world, making up about 38 percent of meat production worldwide Some experts believe the pig is a scavenger and not meant for human consumption. Some experts believe they're considered the garbage and waste eliminators of the farm, often eating literally anything they can find. This includes not only bugs, insects and whatever leftover scraps they find laying around, but also their own feces, as well as the dead carcasses of sick animals, including their own young. Just knowing what a pig's diet is like can explain why the meat of the pig can be so dirty or at the very least not so appetizing to consume.

Reasons to avoid pork:

1. The Pig's Problematic Digestive System:

There are reasons that the meat of the pig becomes more saturated with toxins than many of its counterpart farm animals. The first reason has to do with the digestive system of a pig. A pig digests whatever it eats rather quickly, in up to about four hours. On the other hand, a cow takes a good 24 hours to digest what it's eaten. During the digestive process, animals (including humans) get rid of excess toxins as well as other components of the food eaten that could be dangerous to health. Since the pig's digestive system operates rather basically, many of these toxins remain in its system to be stored in its more than adequate fatty tissues ready for our consumption. Another issue with the pig is that it has very few functional sweat glands and can barely sweat at all. Sweat glands are a tool the body uses to be rid of toxins. This leaves more toxins in the pig's body. When you consume pork meat, you too get all these toxins that weren't eliminated from the pig. None of us needs more toxins in our systems. In fact, we should all do what we can to eliminate and cut down on toxin exposure. One vital way to do this is by choosing what you eat carefully, and for me, that definitely includes completely avoiding pork products of any kind.

2. Increased Cancer Risk from Bacon and Other Processed Pork:

According to the World Health Organization, processed meat like ham, bacon and sausage causes cancer. The International Agency for Research on Cancer actually classifies processed meat as a carcinogen, something that causes cancer. Processed meat is considered to be food items like ham, bacon, sausage, hot dogs and some deli meats. These are mainly pork-derived food products. Unfortunately, pork and processed meat is often consumed by folks following the Atkins and keto diet, for example. Instead, they should be using healthier meat like beef, lamb, bison, or chicken.

3. Swine Flu in Humans:

The swine flu is another virus that has made the leap from pig to human. Influenza or flu viruses can be directly transmitted from pigs to humans, from humans to pigs and from humans to humans. Human infection with flu viruses from pigs are most likely when humans are physically close to infected pigs. Swine influenza virus infections in humans are now being called "variant virus infections in humans." The authorities removed the word "swine." According to the Centers for Disease Control and Prevention, H1N1 and H3N2 are swine flu viruses that are "endemic among pig populations in the United States and something that the industry deals with routinely." Outbreaks can occur year-round. H1N1 has been observed in pig populations since at least 1930, while H3N2 began in the United States around 1998. According to the CDC, swine flu has not been shown to be transmissible to people through eating properly handled and prepared pork. Properly prepared means cooking pork to an internal temperature of 160 degrees F, which is supposed to kill all viruses and other foodborne pathogens.

4. Trichinosis Dangers:

Pigs carry a variety of parasites in their bodies and meat. Some of these parasites are difficult to kill even when cooking. This is the reason there are so many warnings out there about eating undercooked pork. One of the biggest concerns with eating pork meat is trichinosis or trichinellosis. This is an infection that humans get from eating undercooked or uncooked pork that contains the larvae of the *trichinella* worm. In some countries and cultures, they actually consume pork raw. This worm parasite is very commonly found in pork. When the worm, most often living in cysts in the stomach, opens through stomach acids, its larvae are released into the body of the pig. These new worms make their homes in the muscles of the pig. An unknowing human body can consume this infected meat flesh. Similarly, to what these worms do to the pig, they can also do to humans.

If you eat undercooked or raw pork that contains the parasite, then you are also swallowing *trichinella* larvae encased in a cyst. Your digestive juices dissolve the cyst, but that only unleashes the parasite into your insides. The larvae then penetrate your small intestine, where they mature into adult worms and mate. If you're at this stage of trichinosis, you may experience abdominal pain, diarrhea, fatigue, nausea and vomiting. Approximately a week after eating the infected pork, the adult female worms now inside your body produce larvae that enter your bloodstream and eventually burrow into muscle or other tissue. Once this tissue invasion occurs, symptoms of trichinosis include:

a. Headache

b. High fever

c. General weakness

d. Muscle pain and tenderness

e. Pink eye (conjunctivitis)

f. Sensitivity to light

g. Swelling of the eyelids or face

Abdominal symptoms can occur one to two days after infection while additional symptoms usually start two to eight weeks after infection. According to Mayo Clinic, the severity of symptoms typically depends on the number of larvae consumed in the infected meat. The CDC recommends thorough cooking of pork as well as freezing the pork meat prior to cooking to kill off any worms.

5. Pigs Harbor Common Viruses and Parasites:

Pigs carry many viruses and parasites with them. Whether by coming in direct contact with them through farms or by eating their meat, we put ourselves at higher risk of getting one of these painful, often debilitating diseases (not to mention put our bodies on toxic overload).

Pigs are primary carriers of:

a. Taenia solium tapeworm

b. Hepatitis E virus (HEV) — In developed countries, sporadic cases of HEV genotype 3 have occurred in humans after eating uncooked or undercooked pork.

c. Porcine reproductive and respiratory syndrome, aka blue-ear pig disease

d. Nipah virus

e. Menangle virus

f. Viruses in the family Paramyxoviridae

Each of these parasites and viruses can lead to serious health problems that can last for years to come.

6. Factory Farming and Pigs:

Today, ninety seven percent of pigs in the United States are raised in factory farms. This means that these pigs never live a healthy life of fresh air and wide-open pastures. If you're a pork eater, you should know that it's very likely (only 3 percent unlikely) that you're eating the meat of a pig that spent all of its time in a crowded warehouses with no fresh air or exercise, fed a steady diet of harmful drugs to keep the pig breathing as producers make pigs grow faster and fatter. These drugs often cause the pigs to become crippled under their own excessive and unnatural weight gain.

7. Drug Resistant Bacteria in Pork Chops and Ground Pork:

It's estimated that 70 percent of factory-farmed pigs have pneumonia when they go to the slaughterhouse. Unsightly factory-farm conditions of filth and extreme overcrowding lead pigs to have an extreme likelihood for serious diseases. The conditions are so bad that the only way to keep these

pigs barely alive at times is to misuse and overuse antibiotics. Similarly,
to humans, pigs are more commonly developing diseases that are resistant
to antibiotics.

Chapter 3

My Results

I previously indicated that I am not a professional medical practitioner. This chapter is intended to answer the question of why I chose to write and or compile a book about the correlation between nutrition and health without any professional medical educational and or career background.

I am nutritionally consistent, which has been proven by means of medical examination. Apart from freedom of speech, this does to some extent qualify me to share my nutritional practices with others to promote healthy lifestyles. Although I am not a medical practitioner, I can share with others my results and what I did to achieve these results.

In February of 2022 before my 40th birthday in May of 2022, I received my results from my annual physical exam that was conducted at the Henry Ford Hospital here in Detroit, Michigan. Here are my serum and lipoid profile test results:

- 136 mmol / L Sodium: Normal Range: 135 - 145 mmol / L
- My potassium, chloride, carbon dioxide, anion gap, blood urea nitrogen, and creatinine values were all in excellent standing.
- 79 mg / dL Glucose: Normal Range: 60 - 140 mg / dL
- 9.6 mg / dL Calcium: Normal Range: 8.6 - 10.4 mg / dL
- 136 mg / dL total Cholesterol: Normal Range: 120 - 200 mg / dL
- 33 Triglyceride Level: Normal Range: 40 - 200 mg / dL
- 64 mg / dL HDL Cholesterol: Normal Range: less than 40 mg / dL
- 65 mg / dL LDL Cholesterol: Normal Range: 70 - 130 mg / dL
- My VLDL Value: 7

Chapter 4

Momentum

When sharing with others my nutritional practices, some people or readers, some people previously asked me, "Does it really take all of this to be healthy?" The word "healthy" is vague. By this I mean that some people define being healthy as not being diagnosed with any disease while others could possibly define being healthy as how they feel, their physical mobility, no pain, etc.

My response to this question is, "You get out it (your body) what you put into it (your body)." Healthy lifestyle and nutritional practices are like making investments into your body.

When I wrote and compiled the first version of this book titled *7 Years Weight Loss, 7 Years Vegetarian, & 7 Years Organic*, I was not exercising on a consistent basis. During my undergraduate studies, I would exercise off and on. Then from 2013 to 2015, I also exercised off and on. I started to resume exercising in early 2020. Then I was unable to do so.

Then in November of 2020, I joined LA Fitness. Although I was experiencing phenomenal health benefits because of my healthy nutritional practices, I quickly noticed a difference in health benefits I saw when I only ate really healthy versus eating really healthy and consistent exercising. It takes both healthy eating and exercising.

Although my schedule was not conducive for me to schedule training sessions with a personal trainer, I still continue to regularly go to the gym to cardio exercise. I don't want to make any excuses to stop me from exercising.

Personal Trainers are very important. I strongly advise readers to consult a Personal Trainer prior to lifting weights. If a person is not careful, it is possible to incur irreparable damage because of either lifting weight incorrectly or lifting too many weights.

My favorite exercise machine is the Precor Elliptical machine. This machine provides the ideal overall body cardio workout with just the right amount of resistance. I personally prefer exercise facilities or indoor exercise over outdoor exercise. I don't like to exercise outside in the Winter because it is too cold outside, the air is polluted in the summer time, and there is typically no resistance with outdoor exercising. Another reason why I prefer indoor exercise on exercise machines as opposed to outdoor exercising is because machines tend to provide an approximate number of calories burned. Exercise machines can also encourage people to set calories burning goals of calories to be burned within set time frames making their exercise more effective.

In the beginning of chapter 1, I discussed my development of eating patterns. I believe this fundamental concept is very important to nutritional consistency. In order for me to determine my eating pattern, I implemented the "weaning" concept. I started where I was at nutritionally then I gradually weaned myself from unhealthy foods by setting nutritional goals. Although this book provides some helpful nutritional tips and suggests some healthier foods, these are the underlying principle and concepts of this book (eating patterns, gradual weaning, then consistency).

Over time, I personally developed eating and exercise patterns. As time progressed and I continued the same eating and exercise habits, it became easier for me to eat healthy + exercise.

Unfortunately, some people have this pessimistic negative of an addiction to healthy foods. I believe there are good and bad habits.

I believe readers should understand that eating and exercise patterns are developed from habits. It becomes habitual like a pattern. This is why I believe some are able to consistently eat healthy for years because it is largely due to habit.

Some experts even believe that eating patterns or habits began to shape our appetites and the types of foods we crave. For instance, if you were to ask a person who has eaten healthy for several years if they want to go back to eating more unhealthy foods, they would or could probably tell you they don't crave as much junk food. Habitual eating patterns impacts cravings.

This concept is also applicable to exercise. In the beginning, people who start exercising should make the decision to persevere to make exercise habitual.

In my opinion, it is harder in the beginning for a person to convert from constantly eating unhealthy foods to consuming healthier foods.

It seems really hard at first than over time it becomes easier. Momentum builds over years and years of making the right nutritional choices. Then people realize that they don't want to throw away this momentum of healthy eating for an unhealthy snack.

This momentum is further established when people see and feel the physical results of their healthy eating and exercise practices.

Chapter 5

Natural then Mostly Organic

The term "organic" is controversial. I have argued with people primarily regarding the health benefits and costs of organic foods in contrast to conventional foods. All organic implies is the stuff that our parents and grandparents grew up on. They grew up without all of the synthetic preservatives found in foods today.

During my personal weaning process during 2012, I began eating natural foods and incorporated organic foods. Up until this point, I never heard of organic foods. Then I gradually weaned myself to eat foods containing mostly organic ingredients most of time. I don't aim for a specific percentage. However, I try to carefully read ingredient labels to make sure most of the ingredients are organic.

The United States Department of Agriculture has standards for foods and beverages with the organic label. A company can be subjected to fines if a company labels a product organic and it not meet the organic standard.

Organic Labeling Standards

The four categories of labeling based on product composition & the labeling specifications for each are summarized below:

1.   "100 percent organic":

"100 percent organic" can be used to label any product that contains 100 percent organic ingredients (excluding salt and water, which are considered natural). Most raw, unprocessed farm products can be designated "100 percent organic." Likewise, many value-added farm products that have no added ingredients—such as grain flours, rolled oats, etc.—can also be labeled "100 percent organic."

2.   "Organic":

"Organic" can be used to label any product that contains a minimum of 95 percent organic ingredients (excluding salt and water). Up to 5 percent of the ingredients may be nonorganic agricultural products that are not commercially available as organic and/or nonagricultural products that are on the National List.

3.   "Made with Organic ______":

"Made with Organic ______" can be used to label a product that contains at least 70 percent organically produced ingredients (excluding salt and water). There are a number of detailed constraints regarding the ingredients that comprise the nonorganic portion.

4.   Specific Ingredient Listings:

The specific organic ingredients may be listed in the ingredient statement of products containing less than 70 percent organic contents—for example, "Ingredients: water, barley, beans, organic tomatoes, salt."

Producers who market less than $5,000 worth of organic products annually are not required to apply for organic certification. They must, however, comply with the organic production and handling requirements of the regulations, including recordkeeping (records must be kept for at least 3 years). The products from such noncertified operations cannot be used as organic ingredients in processed products produced by another operation; such noncertified products also are not allowed to display the USDA certified organic seal.

We've all heard to stay away from GMOs (Genetically Modified Organisms). A genetically modified organism is any organism whose genetic material has been altered using genetic engineering techniques. GMOs are used to produce many medications and genetically modified foods and are widely used in scientific research and the production of other goods.

Genetically modified crops approved to be grown in the U.S:

1. Corn

2. Soybeans

3. Canola

4. Sugar beets

5. Alfalfa

6. Papaya

7. Yellow "crook neck" squash

8. Zucchini

9. "Arctic" apple

10. "Innate" potato

Health hazards of genetically modified foods:

1.   GM corn and Roundup herbicide cause tumors and organ damage:

rats fed Monsanto's GM corn NK603 and tiny amounts of Roundup herbicide over a two-year period—the longest ever feeding study involving a GM food—developed severe liver and kidney damage, disturbance to pituitary gland function, and hormonal disruption. Additional findings included increased rates of large tumors and premature deaths.

2.   GM-fed pigs suffered severe stomach inflammation and heavier uteri:

A study found that pigs fed GM corn and soy over 22.7 weeks suffered more severe stomach inflammation than pigs fed a non-GMO diet. GM-fed females had on average a 25% heavier uterus than non-GM-fed females, a possible indicator of disease that requires further investigation.

3.   GM corn altered blood biochemistry, damaged organs, and caused potential
      effects on male fertility:

Rats fed the GM corn MON810 for 45 and 91 days showed differences in organ
and body weights and in blood biochemistry, compared with rats fed a non-GMO
variety grown side-by-side in the same conditions. The authors noted that the
changes could indicate "potential adverse health/toxic effects," which needed
further investigation.

5.   GM potatoes caused damage to mice intestines:

Mice fed a diet of GM potatoes showed abnormalities in the cells and structures
of the small intestine, indicating mild damage to the intestines. A control
group of mice fed non-GMO potatoes containing a naturally occurring toxin
showed no abnormalities. The test shows that the toxin does not break down in
digestion, as GMO proponents claim.

6.   GM corn toxin found in blood of pregnant women:

A study conducted in Canada detected significant levels of the insecticidal
corn protein, Cry1Ab, circulating in the blood of pregnant women and in the
blood supply to unborn fetuses. This study again shows that the toxin does
not break down in digestion, as GMO proponents claim.

Environmental hazards of genetically modified crops:

1.   GM crops increase pesticide use:

According to a study published by published by Washington State University
research professor Charles Benbrook, GM crops have increased overall pesticide
use by 404 million pounds from 1996 through 2011.

2.   GM crops creating "superweeds":

The widespread use of glyphosate herbicide used with herbicide tolerant GM
corn, soybeans, canola, and cotton has led to the creation of herbicide
resistant weeds, which now infest 60 million of acres of farmland throughout
the United States.

3.   GM corn harms aquatic insects:

A 2007 published study by Indiana University environmental science professor found that GM corn produced increased mortality and reduced growth in caddisflies, aquatic insects that are a food resource for higher organisms like fish and amphibians.

4.   GMO contamination of organic and non-GMO crops causes hardships for farmers:

Genetically modified crops are passing their transgenes to organic and non-GMO crops and causing farmers added costs and hardships. The risks and the effects of GMO contamination have unfairly burdened organic and non-GMO farmers with extra work, longer hours, and financial insecurity.

When I debated with people regarding this subject matter, their most common response was, "Nothing is truly organic." To a certain extent that is true. For instance, the environment in which the "organic" crop may be grown in inorganic soil unless it is grown inside of a green house. It is possible to utilize organic soil in a green house. In a green house, all environmental factors can be controlled. However, consider an inorganic crop exposed to herbicides and pesticides grown in inorganic soil, exposed to inorganic rainfall, and exposed to inorganic pollution. We all know the dangers and possible health consequences of exposure to herbicides, pesticides, and synthetic preservatives. There are natural herbicides and pesticides and there are synthetic herbicides and pesticides. There are natural preservatives and there are harmful synthetic preservatives.

Organic foods may have higher nutritional value than conventional food, according to some research. The reason: In the absence of pesticides and fertilizers, plants boost their production of the phytochemicals (vitamins and antioxidants) that strengthen their resistance to bugs and weeds. Some studies have linked pesticides in our food to everything from headaches to cancer to birth defects — but many experts maintain that the levels in conventional food are safe for most healthy adults. Even low-level pesticide exposure, however, can be significantly more toxic for fetuses and children (due to their less-developed immune systems) and for pregnant women (it puts added strain on their already taxed organs), according to a report by the National Academy of Sciences. Pesticide contamination isn't as much of a concern in meats and dairy products (animals may consume some pesticides, depending on their diet), but many scientists *are* concerned about the antibiotics being given to most farm animals: Many are the same antibiotics humans rely on, and overuse of these drugs has already enabled bacteria to develop resistance to them, rendering them less effective in fighting infection. Pesticides were also discussed in Chapter 1: The Importance of Nutrition in the Nutrition and Pollution section.

A key word here is artificial and should give you a good indication that something unnatural is in the product. Typically, artificial colors are chemical-based dyes that are used to color food and drinks. Most processed foods, candies, beverages and many condiments contain artificial coloring.

Some examples of harmful artificial colorings, additives and preservatives are:

1. Yellow No. 5 may cause severe asthma symptoms.

2. Studies have shown that Red Dye No. 2: may cause cancer.

3. Blue #1 and Blue #2 (E133): banned in Norway, Finland, and

France. May cause chromosomal damage. Found in candy, cereal, soft drinks, sports drinks and pet foods.

4. Red Dye # 3 (also Red #40 – a more current dye) (E124):

Banned in 1990 after 8 years of debate from use in many foods and cosmetics. This dye continues to be on the market until supplies run out! Has been proven to cause thyroid cancer and chromosomal damage in laboratory animals. May also interfere with brain-nerve transmission. Found in fruit cocktail, maraschino cherries, cherry pie mix, ice cream, candy, bakery products and more!

5. Yellow #6 (E110) and Yellow Tartrazine (E102): Banned in

Norway and Sweden. Increases the number of kidney and adrenal gland tumors in laboratory animals. May cause chromosomal damage. Found in American cheese, macaroni and cheese, candy, carbonated beverages, lemonade and more!

6. High Fructose Corn Syrup: High fructose corn syrup (HFCS) is made from corn starch and offers a sweet flavor. It is popular because it is cheaper to produce than cane sugar. Starch is a simple sugar, and when broken down the end result is corn syrup, which is 100% glucose. Enzymes are then added to the corn syrup, helping convert the glucose into another simple sugar called fructose. In addition to sweet products, it is found in many other types of foods. Yogurts, breads, frozen pizzas, cereal bars, cocktail peanuts, and boxed macaroni and cheese are a few examples where HFCS is found. Because major health risks have exploded in the past few decades with the increasing popularity of easy to grab processed foods, it is thought that HFCS may increase the risk of obesity and type 2 diabetes.

7. Aspartame: Aspartame is a low-calorie sweetener consisting of two amino acids, namely phenylalanine and aspartic acid. Because it is about 200 times sweeter than sugar, very little is required to get a sweet taste. Aspartame is usually found in diet or sugar-free sodas, diet coke, coke zero, jello (and other gelatins), desserts, sugar-free gum, drink mixes, baking goods, table-top sweeteners, cereal, breath mints, pudding, Kool-Aid, iced tea, chewable vitamins, toothpaste. While watching calorie consumption is important, using artificial additives and sweeteners such as aspartame may cause some health risks. Studies have shown that aspartame may elevate blood glucose and increase anxiety.

8. Caramelized sugar syrup

9. Potassium Bromate: Potassium bromate is a common food additive that is used to strengthen bread and cracker dough, helping it rise during baking; however, California and the international cancer agency lists it as a carcinogen. Potassium bromate has been labeled as causing tumors, toxic to

the kidneys and may even cause DNA damage. Though once baked, it converts to potassium bromide which has been deemed as non-carcinogenic, some residues exist. It has been banned in the United Kingdom, European Union and Canada in food, but the United States still allows it to be added to flour. Labels typically reference it as potassium bromate. Alternatives: bromates, calcium bromate, potassium bromate, sodium bromate, bromated flour.

10. Monosodium Glutamate (MSG): It is no surprise that MSG is on the list. MSG is created by a naturally occurring chemical called glutamate and looks similar to salt or sugar crystals. While glutamate is tasteless, it has the ability to enhance flavors. It is typically found in Chinese food, canned foods, and processed meats. MSG has the GRAS Classification by the Food & Drug Administration which means it is "generally recognized as safe." But due to the controversy surrounding MSG, the FDA requires that it be listed on the label. MSG has gotten a bad rap for years, with numerous claims in late 1960s alleging that food prepared with MSG at Chinese restaurants made people sick; however, many studies report difficulty in finding concrete evidence that there is a problem with MSG. At the same time, some reports have indicated numerous reactions such as headaches, flushing, sweating, facial pressure or tightness, numbness, tingling or burning in the face, neck and other areas, rapid, heart palpitations, chest pain, nausea, and weakness. Labels typically note it as monosodium glutamate or MSG, but it may be disguised by other ingredients that contain MSG such as hydrolyzed soy protein and autolyzed yeast. Alternative names: sodium glutamate, MSG, Accent, Zest, Ajinomoto, and Vetsin.

11. Sodium Benzoate: Sodium benzoate is a common food preservative used in many processed food products and drinks to prevent spoilage. Sodium benzoate is the sodium salt of benzoic acid. It is used as an antifungal preservative in pharmaceutical preparations and foods. Sodium benzoate is often added to acidic food products such as sauerkraut, jellies and jams, and hot sauces; however, some foods, like cranberries, cinnamon, prunes and apples, naturally contain it. It has been suggested that it may help treat hyperammonemia in terms of medication. Concerns have been raised regarding it as a possible cause of hyperactivity in some children, though more studies

are needed according to The European Food Safety Authority. Food labels typically reference it as sodium benzoate. Alternative names: benzoic acid, potassium benzoate, and benzoate.

12. Sodium Sulfite (E221): Preservative used in wine-making and other processed foods. According to the FDA, approximately one in 100 people is sensitive to sulfites in food. The majority of these individuals are asthmatic, suggesting a link between asthma and sulfites. Individuals who are sulfite sensitive may experience headaches, breathing problems, and rashes. In severe cases, sulfites can actually cause death by closing down the airway altogether, leading to cardiac arrest. Found in wine and dried fruit.

13. Sulfur Dioxide (E220): Sulfur additives are toxic and in the United States of America, the Food and Drug Administration have prohibited their use on raw fruit and vegetables. Adverse reactions include bronchial problems, particularly in those prone to asthma, hypotension (low blood pressure), flushing, tingling sensations or anaphylactic shock. It also destroys vitamins B1 and E. Not recommended for consumption by children. The International Labor Organization says to avoid E220 if you suffer from conjunctivitis, bronchitis, emphysema, bronchial asthma, or cardiovascular disease. Found in beer, soft drinks, dried fruit, juices, cordials, wine, vinegar, and potato products.

14. Propyl Paraben: Propyl paraben is commonly used as a preservative in many foods including tortillas, bread products and food dyes; and cross contamination has led to propyl paraben showing up in beverages, dairy products, meat and vegetables. It is commonly found in many cosmetics, such as creams, lotions, shampoos and bath products. A federal study showed that 91 percent of Americans tested had propyl paraben in their urine. This is of concern since propyl paraben is an endocrine-disrupting chemical that is "Generally Recognized as Safe." Studies indicate that subjects had decreased sperm counts and testosterone levels. Additionally, it has been shown to alter the expression of genes, including those in breast cancer cells and to accelerate the growth of breast cancer cells. Harvard School of Public Health shared the results of a recent study linking propyl paraben to impaired

fertility in women. Look for propyl paraben on the food labels to avoid it. Alternative names: 4-Hydroxybenzoesäurepropylester; propyl paraben; propyl p-hydroxybenzoate; propyl parahydroxybenzoate; nipasol; E216

15. BHA And BHT (E320): Butylated hydroxyanisole (BHA) and butylated hydroxytoluene (BHT) are preservatives found in cereals, chewing gum, potato chips, and vegetable oils. This common preservative keeps foods from changing color, changing flavor or becoming rancid. Affects the neurological system of the brain, alters behavior and has a potential to cause cancer. BHA and BHT are oxidants which form cancer-causing reactive compounds in your body. Found in potato chips, gum, cereal, frozen sausages, enriched rice, lard, shortening, candy, jello.

Another argument I heard once was, "You don't know that it is truly organic unless you monitored the production process or unless you were present to see the company make the product." This is why I read the ingredient labels. If the company is marketing a product as organic that is not truly organic, then I will hold this company accountable once I am aware of this.

One of the benefits I appreciate about organic products are their ingredient labels being easier read. Reading ingredient labels is important. As a consumer, I appreciate the transparency of companies who produce organic products.

Organic foods can be easier to digest and if the foods are healthy the body will be busy absorbing the nutrients as the food works its way through the body. The human digestion system is not as simple as chewing food and then sending it to the stomach. Food encounters a variety of areas within the body before it is eventually discarded as waste, and in each step of the digestive process there is the potential for conventionally produced foods to invade the body with toxins. Organic foods do not have this same potential detrimental effect on the human body.

1. The Mouth: Food enters the body through the mouth where it is chewed and broken down with the help of saliva. Foods that are not organic, and

which are potentially tainted with toxic chemicals and artificial preservatives, begin their assault on the body in this step.

2. The Esophagus and Stomach: Food is sent down to the stomach via the esophagus. In both areas, any toxins within conventionally produced foods are being absorbed into the body.

3. The Small and Large Intestines: All food must make its way through both the small and large intestines before eventually being discarded as waste. Healthy, organic foods will contain the nutrients the body needs and will be utilized by the body accordingly. Foods that are unhealthy, or foods that contain the various chemicals sometimes used in the production of some conventional foods, may be harder for the body to digest and may have detrimental effects on the body.

The next argument I have debated is the price difference between organic, natural, and conventional products. I was often asked is the price difference justified. Some organic products costs only $1.00 or $2.00 more than their conventional counterparts. It all depends on what you purchase. In life, you typically get what you pay for. I want consumers to understand that companies who produce organic products are in a business. I want consumers to understand that these companies who produce organic products incur extra costs to avoid adding harmful antibiotics, steroids, additives, and preservatives into the foods, beverages, and other organic or natural products we purchase. I want consumers to understand and appreciate the farmers who grow organic crops and the companies who produce organic and natural products. We can show our appreciation by patronizing these farmers and companies on a consistent basis instead of complaining about the price difference. Yes, the price difference is justified!

I was also often asked, "Do you feel different?" My response has always been, "Yes, because I do it consistently." Internally I do feel a difference. I feel that my blood and internal organs are clean, purified. I know I am in good health.

I personally select foods and beverages (apart from water) that are mostly organic or contains a substantial amount of organic ingredients. I utilize organic liquid soap, organic or natural deodorant, and natural toothpaste. I really would like to try the organic and or natural brand of cosmetics produced by Ecco Bella. Ecco Bella offers a line of organic cosmetics.

Some people want to do everything organic. They want organic laundry detergent. Organic fabric and or organic clothing. They want only organic cleaning products. Yes, organic cleaning products are good. However, there are some strains of bacteria that only chlorine (bleach) can kill. Yet, there are some bacteria chlorine cannot kill.

However, we should try to use as much natural cleaning products as possible. A lot of us have at one point mixed too much dish detergent with the bleach or another cleaner with something else. Conventional cleaning products tend to be carcinogenic or contain a lot of carcinogens. Some experts encourage consumers to make their own cleaning products at home or to purchase more natural cleaning products.

The average household contains about 62 toxic chemicals, say environmental experts. We're exposed to them routinely — from the phthalates in synthetic fragrances to the noxious fumes in oven cleaners. Ingredients in common household products have been linked to asthma, cancer, reproductive disorders, hormone disruption and neurotoxicity.

1. Phthalates

Found in: Many fragranced household products, such as air fresheners, dish soap, even toilet paper. Because of proprietary laws, companies don't have to disclose what's in their scents, so you won't find phthalates on a label. If you see the word "fragrance" on a label, there's a good chance phthalates are present.

Health Risks: Phthalates are known endocrine disruptors. Men with higher phthalate compounds in their blood had correspondingly reduced sperm counts, according to a 2003 study conducted by researchers from the Centers for Disease

Control and Prevention and the Harvard School of Public Health. Although exposure to phthalates mainly occurs through inhalation, it can also happen through skin contact with scented soaps, which is a significant problem. Unlike the digestive system, the skin has no safeguards against toxins. Absorbed chemicals go straight to organs.

2.   Perchloroethylene or "PERC"

Found in: Dry-cleaning solutions, spot removers, and carpet and upholstery cleaners.

Health Risks: Perc is a neurotoxin, according to the chief scientist of environmental protection for the New York Attorney General's office. And the EPA classifies perc as a "possible carcinogen" as well. People who live in residential buildings where dry cleaners are located have reported dizziness, loss of coordination and other symptoms. While the EPA has ordered a phase-out of perc machines in residential buildings by 2020, California is going even further and plans to eliminate all use of perc by 2023 because of its suspected health risks. The route of exposure is most often inhalation: that telltale smell on clothes when they return from the dry cleaner, or the fumes that linger after cleaning carpets.

3.   Triclosan

Found in: Most liquid dishwashing detergents and hand soaps labeled "antibacterial."

Health Risks: Triclosan is an aggressive antibacterial agent that can promote the growth of drug-resistant bacteria. The American Medical Association has found no evidence that these antimicrobials make us healthier or safer, and they're particularly concerned because they don't want us overusing antibacterial chemicals — that's how microbes develop resistance, and not just to these [household antibacterial], but also to real antibiotics that we need. Other studies have now found dangerous concentrations of triclosan in rivers and streams, where it is toxic to algae. The EPA is currently investigating whether triclosan may also disrupt endocrine (hormonal) function. It is a probable carcinogen. At press time, the agency was reviewing the safety of triclosan in consumer products.

4.   Quarternary Ammonium Compounds, or "QUATS"

Found in: Fabric softener liquids and sheets, most household cleaners labeled "antibacterial."

Health Risks: Quats are another type of antimicrobial, and thus pose the same problem as triclosan by helping breed antibiotic-resistant bacteria. They're also a skin irritant; one 10-year study of contact dermatitis found quats to be one of the leading causes. They're also suspected as a culprit for respiratory disorders. There's evidence that even healthy people who are [exposed to quats] on a regular basis develop asthma as a result.

5.   2-Butoxyethanol

Found in: Window, kitchen and multipurpose cleaners.

Health Risks: 2-butoxyethanol is the key ingredient in many window cleaners and gives them their characteristic sweet smell. It belongs in the category of "glycol ethers," a set of powerful solvents that don't mess around. Law does not require 2-butoxyethanol to be listed on a product's label. According to the EPA's Web site, in addition to causing sore throats when inhaled, at high levels glycol ethers can also contribute to narcosis, pulmonary edema, and severe liver and kidney damage. The EPA (Environmental Protection Agency) sets a standard on 2-butoxyethanol for workplace safety. If you're cleaning at home in a confined area, like an unventilated bathroom, you can actually end up getting 2-butoxyethanol in the air at levels that are higher than workplace safety standards.

6.   Ammonia

Found in: Polishing agents for bathroom fixtures, sinks and jewelry; also, in glass cleaner.

Health Risks: Because ammonia evaporates and doesn't leave streaks, it's another common ingredient in commercial window cleaners. That sparkle has a price. Ammonia is a powerful irritant. It's going to affect you right away. The people who will be really affected are those who have asthma, and elderly people with lung issues and breathing problems. It's almost always inhaled. People who get a lot of ammonia exposure, like housekeepers, will often develop chronic bronchitis and asthma." Ammonia can also create a poisonous gas if it's mixed with bleach.

7.   Sodium Hydroxide

Found in: Oven cleaners and drain openers.

Health Risks: Otherwise known as lye, sodium hydroxide is extremely corrosive: If it touches your skin or gets in your eyes, it can cause severe burns. Routes of exposure are skin contact and inhalation. Inhaling sodium hydroxide can cause a sore throat that lasts for days.

Last but not least, I wanted to briefly discuss organic junk foods. We are all familiar with junk food, which are inclusive of chips, candy bars, soda, etc. A lot of people have this misconception that just because they consume junk food with an organic food label, they are eating healthy. This is not true. Although the organic candy bar may be healthier for you, because it does not contain all of the typical synthetic preservatives in the conventional candy bar, it is still not considered a healthy food. You want to eat healthy foods.

Chapter 6

Organic and Natural Supplements

UPDATE:

I remembered the advice of one of my Mother's friends who was or is still a RN or Registered Nurse. My Mother's friend suggested consumption of vitamins and or supplements at night time right before going to sleep. The reason being is that vitamins and or supplements supposedly taken at night immediately before sleep are better absorbed by the body due less internal bodily processes that normally occurs during day time hours.

Half of all-American adults—including 70 percent of those age 65 and older—take a multivitamin or another vitamin or mineral supplement regularly. The total price tag exceeds $12 billion per year. Some experts believe it is nearly impossible for all of our daily nutritional needs to be met from food. They believe this to be especially true for vegetarians and vegans. I personally try to get my most of my protein if not all of it and fibers from the foods I consume. As a vegetarian, I take a multi-vitamin and calcium supplement daily.

However, some experts believe otherwise. According to the findings of extensive research conducted by John Hopkins University, multivitamins did not reduce risk for heart disease, cancer, and cognitive decline. This study also suggested higher dosages of vitamin E and beta carotene are harmful. They believe pills are not a shortcut to better health and prevention of chronic diseases. They argue there is stronger evidence of benefits attributed to a healthy diet, maintaining a healthy weight, reducing saturated and trans-fats, reducing sodium, and reducing sugar.

Some experts believe supplements can plug dietary gaps, but nutrients from food are most important. These experts believe you should try to improve your diet before turning to supplements. They believe food contains nutrients, such as flavonoids and antioxidants that aren't in most supplements. They believe that the most potent nutrients come from food. Some experts believe as we get older, our ability to absorb nutrients from food decreases. Also, our energy needs aren't the same, and we tend to eat less. Some believe even if you eat a healthy, well-balanced diet, you may still fall short of needed nutrients.

To counteract oxidative stress, the body produces an armory of antioxidants to defend itself. However, your body's internal production of antioxidants is not enough to neutralize all the free radicals. This is why some experts also believe vitamins and supplements are necessary for overall health.

A nutrient is anything that provides nourishment essential for growth and the maintenance of life. This includes micronutrients and macronutrients. Fatty acids and amino acids are also nutrients. Vitamins and minerals are the two types of micronutrients. While only needed in small amounts, they play important roles in human development and well-being, including the regulation of metabolism, heartbeat, cellular pH, and bone density. Lack of micronutrients can lead to stunted growth in children and increased risk for various diseases in adulthood. Without proper consumption of micronutrients, humans can suffer from diseases such as rickets (lack of vitamin D), scurvy (lack of vitamin C), and osteoporosis (lack of calcium). Vitamins are available in two forms: water-soluble and fat-soluble. Water-soluble vitamins are easily lost through bodily fluids and must be replaced each day. Water-soluble vitamins include the B-complex vitamins and vitamin C. Vitamins B6 and B12 are two of the most well-known B-complex vitamins. Since they are not lost as easily as their water-soluble counterparts, fat-soluble vitamins tend to accumulate within the body and are not needed on a daily basis. The fat-soluble vitamins are A, D, E and K.

The three macronutrients all have their own specific roles and functions in the body and supply us with calories or energy. For this reason, the body requires these nutrients in relatively large amounts to grow, develop, repair and feel good! Each macronutrient is almost always found in every item of food. As an example, the nutritional composition of an avocado is generally made up of 75% (good) fats, 20% carbohydrates and 5% protein, therefore this is clearly a fat-based food. On the other hand, a banana consists of 95%

carbohydrates, with only small amounts of protein and fats. Healthy fats are an essential part of a healthy diet and should account for about 15-20% what you consume. They help by improving brain development, overall cell functioning, protecting the body's organs and even helping you absorb vitamins found in foods. Protein is essential for repairing and regenerating body tissues and cells, a healthy functioning immune system and manufacturing hormones. This wouldn't be possible without amino acids, which are found in protein-based foods. In total there are 20 types of amino acids, 9 of which are 'essential' and can only be found in certain foods. Good sources of protein: Beans, pulses and legumes, seeds (hemp, chia, flax), nuts (unsalted), quinoa, avocado, beets, raw greens (kale, spinach). Carbohydrates are comprised of small chains of sugar which the digestive body breaks down into glucose to use as the body's primarily energy source and therefore need to make up around 45-65% of a diet.

List of nutrients:

1.   Water:
Hydration is very important. Our bodies are comprised of up to 60 percent water. Several days without water can lead to serious illness and possibly death. Water is critical for waste removal, temperature regulation, and it is an essential element for every cell. You should drink water throughout the day, eat fruits and vegetables that consists of water, and minimize coffee, sugar, and carbonated beverages.

2. Carbohydrates:
Carbohydrates or carbs are broken down into glucose, which is your brain and body's main fuel. Some experts believe carbs also ensure our bodies are not breaking down proteins to gain energy, preventing loss of muscle mass. Complex carbohydrates take longer to digest and helps keep you fuller for a longer period of time. This should enable you to reduce unhealthy snacking. Vegetables and fruits are examples of complex carbohydrates.

3. Protein-Amino Acids:
Protein is essential in forming muscles to creating new enzymes and hormones. Proteins are comprised of small building blocks called amino

acids. There are twenty amino acids in total, but the nine essential amino acids are:

    a. Histidine

    b. Isoleucine

    c. Leucine

    d. Lysine

    e. Methionine

    f. Phenylalanine

    g. Threonine

    h. Tryptophan

    i. Valine

Animal proteins are believed to provide all essential amino acids, while plant proteins may lack several of these essential elements. Experts recommend including a variety of proteins in your diet such as lean meat, eggs, diary, nuts, and beans.

4. Fat:

Unsaturated fat is an essential nutrient that boosts absorption of vitamins and helps protect organs. Good sources of unsaturated fat include: avocados, nuts, and salmon.

5. Vitamins:

A vitamin is an organic compound and an essential micronutrient that the body needs in small amounts. The essential vitamins are:

    a. Vitamin A:

    b. B Vitamins

    c. Vitamin C

    d. Vitamin D: especially important for bone growth, cardiovascular, health, nervous system health, and immune health

    e. Vitamin E

6. Minerals:

Minerals are micronutrients. Minerals are also available in two forms: macrominerals and microminerals. Macrominerals are needed in larger amounts and include the following:

a. Calcium: 99% of the body's calcium is found in our bones and

   teeth

b. Magnesium

c. Phosphorus

   d. Sodium: keeps nerves and muscles working correctly (moderate consumption recommended)

e. Potassium

Microminerals are only needed in trace amounts and include the following:

a. Iron

b. Copper

c. Iodine

d. Zinc

e. Fluoride

Electrolytes are minerals in body fluids. They include sodium, potassium, magnesium, and chloride. When you are dehydrated, your body does not have enough fluid and electrolytes.

7. Omega 3-Fatty Acids:

It has been proven that omega-3 fatty acids optimize brain health and possibly aid in the function of the heart. Unlike fatty acids, your body cannot create omega-3. It is crucial for you to get your omega-3 intake from your diet. Salmon, mackerel, and sardines contain active omega-3 fatty acids, which requires no conversion. Plant based sources include chia seeds, flax, and walnuts. These foods contain an inactive form of omega-3 that your body has to convert before it can use, and only in small amounts. You can also take fish oil or algae-based supplements.

Macrominerals

Major minerals

Mineral	Function	Sources
Sodium	Needed for proper fluid balance, nerve transmission, and muscle contraction	Table salt, soy sauce; large amounts in processed foods; small amounts in milk, vegetables, and unprocessed meats
Chloride	Needed for proper fluid balance, stomach acid	Table salt, soy sauce; large amounts in processed foods; small amounts in milk, meats, and vegetables
	Needed for proper fluid balance, nerve	

Potassium	transmission, and muscle contraction	Meats, milk, fresh fruits and vegetables, legumes
Calcium	Important for healthy bones and teeth; helps muscles relax and contract; important in nerve functioning, blood clotting, blood pressure regulation, immune system health	Milk and milk products; canned fish with bones (salmon, sardines); fortified tofu and fortified soy milk; greens (broccoli, mustard greens); legumes
Phosphorus	Important for healthy bones and teeth; found in every cell; part of the system that maintains acid-base balance	Meat, fish, poultry, eggs, milk, processed foods (including soda pop)

Magnesium	Found in bones; needed for making protein, muscle contraction, nerve transmission, immune system health	Nuts and seeds; legumes; leafy, green vegetables; seafood; chocolate; artichokes; "hard" drinking water
Sulfur	Found in protein molecules	Occurs in foods as part of protein: meats, poultry, fish, eggs, milk, legumes, nuts

Trace minerals (microminerals)

Mineral	Function	Sources
Iron	Part of a molecule (hemoglobin) found in red blood cells that carries oxygen in the body; needed for energy metabolism	Organ meats; red meats; fish; poultry; shellfish (especially clams); egg yolks; legumes; dried fruits; dark, leafy greens
	Part of many enzymes; needed for making protein and genetic material; has a function in taste perception, wound healing, normal fetal development, production of sperm, normal growth and	

Zinc	sexual maturation, immune system health	Meats, fish, poultry, vegetables
Iodine	Found in thyroid hormone, which helps regulate growth, development, and metabolism	Seafood, foods grown in iodine-rich soil, iodized salt, bread, dairy products
Selenium	Antioxidant	Meats, seafood,
Copper	Part of many enzymes; needed for iron metabolism	Legumes, nuts and seeds, organ meats, drinking water
		Widespread in foods, especially plant foods

Manganese	Part of many enzymes	
Fluoride	Involved in formation of bones and teeth; helps prevent tooth decay	Drinking water (either fluoridated or naturally containing fluoride), fish, and most teas
Chromium	Works closely with insulin to regulate blood sugar (glucose) levels	Unrefined foods, especially liver, brewer's yeast, nuts, cheeses
		Legumes; leafy greens; leafy,

		green vegetables; milk; liver
Molybdenum	Part of some enzymes	

Other trace nutrients known to be essential in tiny amounts include nickel, silicon, vanadium, and cobalt.

Minerals further explained:

1. Calcium:

    Your body needs calcium to build strong bones and teeth. Calcium also plays a role in nerve transmissions, muscle function -- including that of the heart -- and hormone secretion. The Institute of Medicine recommends adults consume 1,000 to 1,200 milligrams of calcium per day. Good sources of calcium include dairy products like milk and yogurt and vegetables like kale, broccoli and cabbage. Too much calcium can clog your arteries.

2. Potassium:

    Potassium controls the electrical activity of your heart, making it vital to maintaining a normal heart rhythm. Your body also needs it to build proteins, break down and use carbohydrates, maintain the pH balance of the blood and support normal growth. Adults should consume 4,700 milligrams of potassium per day, according to the Institute of Medicine. Many foods contain potassium, including beef, fish, chicken, cantaloupe, potatoes, tomatoes and lima beans.

3. Sodium:

    Although too much sodium can increase your risk for developing high blood pressure, your body needs sodium to stimulate nerve and muscle function, maintain the correct balance of fluid in the cells and support the absorption of other nutrients including chloride, amino acids and glucose. Your body only requires 180 to 500 milligrams of sodium per day, but the Institute of Medicine sets the adequate intake, the amount expected to meet or exceed normal circulating nutrient values, at 1,500 milligrams per day. To avoid health problems, the Dietary Guidelines for Americans suggests limiting your sodium intake to no more than 2,300 milligrams per day, and those over 51 or with certain health conditions should consume no more than the listed adequate intake of 1,500 milligrams.

4. Magnesium:

Your body needs magnesium to support more than 300 biochemical reactions. Magnesium supports muscle and nerve function, keeps your heart beating regularly, builds strong bones and boosts immunity. The Institute of Medicine recommends adult women consume 310 to 320 milligrams per day, while men need 400 to 420 milligrams per day. Beans, nuts, and green vegetables serve as good sources of magnesium.

5. Phosphorus:

Phosphorus plays an important role in building strong bones and teeth, producing proteins the body needs and repairing cells. Adult men and women should consume 700 milligrams of phosphorus a day, according to the Institute of Medicine. Dairy food and meat contribute phosphorus to your diet.

6. Chloride:

Chloride usually consumed as a salt compound such as sodium chloride -- better known as table salt -- balances the fluids in your body and plays an essential role in the production of digestive juices in the stomach. With the high salt content of foods, most people meet the daily recommended intake of 1,800 to 2,300 milligrams per day.

7. Trace Minerals:

Trace minerals, those minerals your body only needs in small amounts, also support important bodily functions. Your body uses iron to produce hemoglobin and myoglobin, proteins that carry oxygen in your body. The production of thyroid hormones that regulate nearly every cell in the body requires iodine. Manganese regulates blood sugar, enhances the absorption of calcium and plays a role in the production of connective tissues and bones. Chromium enhances the action of insulin making it important in regulating blood sugar. Fluoride keeps your teeth strong and healthy. Your body needs copper, selenium, molybdenum and zinc to produce enzymes important in various reactions throughout the body.

Vitamins are substances that your body needs to grow and develop normally. Vitamins are nutrients your body needs to function and fight off disease. There are 13 vitamins that are essential to your body working well. Knowledge of the different types and understanding the purpose of these vitamins are important for good health. There are two types of vitamins: fat-soluble and water-soluble. Fat-soluble vitamins are stored in your fat cells, consequently requiring fat in order to be absorbed. Water-soluble vitamins are not stored in your body; therefore, they need to be replenished daily. Your body takes what it needs from the food you eat and then excretes what is not needed as waste. Here is a list of some vitamin types and common food sources:

Fat-Soluble Vitamins:

1. Vitamin A - comes from orange colored fruits and vegetables; dark leafy greens, like kale

2. Vitamin D - can be found in fortified milk and dairy products; cereals; (and of course, sunshine!)

3. Vitamin E - is found in leafy green vegetables; seeds; nuts

4. Vitamin K - can be found in dark green leafy vegetables; turnip/beet greens

Water-Soluble Vitamins:

1. Vitamin B1, or Thiamin - come from liver; nuts; seeds

2. Vitamin B2, or Riboflavin - comes from dairy products

3. Vitamin B3, or Niacin - comes from meat; fish; poultry

4. Vitamin B5, or Pantothenic Acid - comes from meat; poultry

5. Vitamin B6, or Pyridoxine - comes from soy products

6. Vitamin B7, or Biotin - is found in fruits; meats

7. Vitamin B9, or Folic Acid (Folate) - comes from leafy vegetables

8. Vitamin B12 - comes from fish; poultry; meat; dairy products

9. Vitamin C - comes from citrus fruits and juices, such as oranges and grapefruits; red, yellow, and green peppers

Vitamins are used in many different ways inside your body.

While vitamins do not directly serve as a source of energy, they do help the enzymes that generate energy from nutrients such as carbohydrates and fats.

Purposes of vitamins:

1.   Vitamin A:
    One of vitamin A's main roles is in the production of retinal. Your body uses retinal in the rods and cones of your eyes to sense light and help prevent night blindness. Vitamin A is also important for your teeth, bones, skin, reproduction, and a healthy immune system.

2.   B Complex Vitamins:

    The B complex vitamins include thiamin (B1), riboflavin (B2), niacin (B3), pantothenic acid (B5), pyridoxine (B6), biotin (B7), folic acid (B9), and B12. They serve many purposes in your body, including aiding in energy production, making red blood cells, and making new DNA so cells can multiply. They are also required for healthy nerve and brain function, intestinal health, and cardiovascular health.

3.   Vitamin C:
    Vitamin C, an antioxidant, may help prevent cell damage and reduce risk for certain cancers, heart disease, and other diseases. Vitamin C is vital to the formation of collagen, which keeps your blood vessels strong and holds your teeth in their sockets. In addition, vitamin C is important to wound healing and helping your body absorb iron.

You can usually get all your vitamins from the foods you eat. Your body can also make vitamins D and K. People who eat a vegetarian diet may need to take a vitamin B12 supplement. Each vitamin has specific jobs. If you have low levels of certain vitamins, you may get health problems. For example, if you don't get enough vitamin C, you could become anemic. Some vitamins may help prevent medical problems. Vitamin A prevents night blindness. The best way to get enough vitamins is to eat a balanced diet with a variety of foods. In some cases, you may need to take vitamin supplements. It's a good idea to ask your health care provider first.

Some people justify higher intake of vitamins due to lower absorption rates and their bodies producing less antioxidants over time. High doses of some vitamins can cause problems.

VITAMIN	BENEFITS	RECOMMENDED AMOUNT (daily RDA* or daily AI**)	UPPER LIMIT (UL) per day
RETINOIDS AND CAROTENE (vitamin A; includes retinol, retinal, retinyl esters, and retinoic acid and are also referred to as "preformed" vitamin A. Beta carotene can easily be converted to vitamin A as needed.)	Essential for vision Lycopene may lower prostate cancer risk. Keeps tissues and skin healthy. Plays an important role in bone growth and in the immune system. Diets rich in the carotenoids alpha carotene and lycopene seem to lower lung cancer risk. Carotenoids act as antioxidants. Foods rich in the carotenoids lutein and zeaxanthin may	M: 900 mcg (3,000 IU) W: 700 mcg (2,333 IU) Some supplements report vitamin A in international units (IU's).	3,000 mcg (about 10,000 IU)

	protect against cataracts		
THIAMIN (vitamin B_1)	Helps convert food into energy. Needed for healthy skin, hair, muscles, and brain and is critical for nerve function.	M: 1.2 mg, W: 1.1 mg	Not known
RIBOFLAVIN (vitamin B_2)	Helps convert food into energy. Needed for healthy skin, hair, blood, and brain	M: 1.3 mg, W: 1.1 mg	Not known
NIACIN (vitamin B_3, nicotinic acid)	Helps convert food into energy. Essential for healthy skin, blood cells, brain, and nervous system	M: 16 mg, W: 14 mg	35 mg

| PANTOTHENIC ACID (vitamin B_5) | Helps convert food into energy. Helps make lipids (fats), neurotransmitters, steroid hormones, and hemoglobin | M: 5 mg, W: 5 mg | Not known |
| PYRIDOXINE (vitamin B_6, pyridoxal, pyridoxine, pyridoxamine) | Aids in lowering homocysteine levels and may reduce the risk of heart disease. Helps convert tryptophan to niacin and serotonin, a neurotransmitter that plays key roles in sleep, appetite, and moods. Helps make red blood cells Influences cognitive | 31-50 years old: M: 1.3 mg, W: 1.3 mg; 51+ years old: M: 1.7 mg, W: 1.5 mg | 100 mg |

	abilities and immune function		
COBALAMIN (vitamin B₁₂)	Aids in lowering homocysteine levels and may lower the risk of heart disease. Assists in making new cells and breaking down some fatty acids and amino acids. Protects nerve cells and encourages their normal growth Helps make red blood cells and DNA	M: 2.4 mcg, W: 2.4 mcg	Not known
BIOTIN	Helps convert food into energy and synthesize glucose. Helps make and break down some fatty	M: 30 mcg, W: 30 mcg	Not known

acids. Needed for healthy bones and hair

| ASCORBIC ACID (vitamin C) | Foods rich in vitamin C may lower the risk for some cancers, including those of the mouth, esophagus, stomach, and breast. Long-term use of supplemental vitamin C may protect against cataracts. Helps make collagen, a connective tissue that knits together wounds and supports blood vessel walls. Helps make the neurotransmitters serotonin and norepinephrine | M: 90 mg, W: 75 mg Smokers: Add 35 mg | 2,000 mg |

	Acts as an antioxidant, neutralizing unstable molecules that can damage cells. Bolsters the immune system		
CHOLINE	Helps make and release the neurotransmitter acetylcholine, which aids in many nerve and brain activities. Plays a role in metabolizing and transporting fats	M: 550 mg, W: 425 mg	3,500 mg
CALCIFEROL (vitamin D)	Helps maintain normal blood levels of calcium and phosphorus, which	31-70: 15 mcg (600 IU) 71+: 20 mcg (800 IU)	50 mcg (2,000 IU)

	strengthen bones. Helps form teeth and bones. Supplements can reduce the number of non-spinal fractures		
ALPHA-TOCOPHEROL (vitamin E)	Acts as an antioxidant, neutralizing unstable molecules that can damage cells. Protects vitamin A and certain lipids from damage. Diets rich in vitamin E may help prevent Alzheimer's disease.	M: 15 mg, W: 15 mg (15 mg equals about 22 IU from natural sources of vitamin E and 33 IU from synthetic vitamin E)	1,000 mg (nearly 1,500 IU natural vitamin E; 2,200 IU synthetic)
FOLIC ACID (vitamin B_9, folate, folacin)	Vital for new cell creation. Helps prevent brain and spine birth defects	M: 400 mcg, W: 400 mcg	1,000 mcg

when taken
early in
pregnancy;
should be taken
regularly by
all women of
child-bearing
age since women
may not know
they are
pregnant in the
first weeks of
pregnancy. Can
lower levels of
homocysteine
and may reduce
heart disease
risk May reduce
risk for colon
cancer. Offsets
breast cancer
risk among
women who
consume alcohol

| PHYLLOQUINONE, MENADIONE (vita min K) | Activates proteins and calcium essential to blood clotting. May help | M: 120 mcg, W: 90 mcg | Not known |

prevent hip
fractures

MINERAL	BENEFITS	RECOMMENDED AMOUNT (daily RDA* or daily AI**)	UPPER LIMIT (UL) per day
CALCIUM	Builds and protects bones and teeth. Helps with muscle contractions and relaxation, blood clotting, and nerve impulse transmission. Plays a role in hormone secretion and enzyme activation. Helps maintain healthy blood pressure	31-50: M: 1,000 mg, W: 1,000 mg 51-70: M: 1,000 mg, W: 1,200 mg, 71+: M: 1,200 mg, W: 1,200 mg	2,500 mg
CHLORIDE	Balances fluids in the body. A	14-50: M/W: 2.3 g, 51-70 M/W:	Not known

	component of stomach acid, essential to digestion	2.0 g, 71+: M/W: 1.8 g	
CHROMIUM	Enhances the activity of insulin, helps maintain normal blood glucose levels, and is needed to free energy from glucose	14-50: M: 35 mcg, 14-18: W: 24 mcg 19-50: W: 25 mcg 51+: M: 30 mcg, W: 20 mcg	Not known
COPPER	Plays an important role in iron metabolism and immune system. Helps make red blood cells	M: 900 mcg, W: 900 mcg	10,000 mcg
FLUORIDE	Encourages strong bone formation. Keeps dental cavities from starting or worsening	M: 4 mg, W: 3 mg	10 mg

IODINE	Part of thyroid hormone, which helps set body temperature and influences nerve and muscle function, reproduction, and growth. Prevents goiter and a congenital thyroid disorder	M: 150 mcg, W: 150 mcg	1,100 mcg
IRON	Helps hemoglobin in red blood cells and myoglobin in muscle cells ferry oxygen throughout the body. Needed for chemical reactions in the body and for making amino acids, collagen, neurotransmitte	19-50: M: 8 mg, W: 18 mg 51+: M: 8 mg, W: 8 mg	45 mg

	rs, and hormones		
MAGNESIUM	Needed for many chemical reactions in the body Works with calcium in muscle contraction, blood clotting, and regulation of blood pressure. Helps build bones and teeth	18+: M: 420 mg, W: 320 mg	350 mg (Note: This upper limit applies to supplements and medicines, such as laxatives, not to dietary magnesium.)
MANGANESE	Helps form bones. Helps metabolize amino acids, cholesterol, and carbohydrates	M: 2.3 mg, W: 1.8 mg	11 mg
MOLYBDENUM	Part of several enzymes, one of which helps	M: 45 mcg, W: 45 mcg	2,000 mcg

	ward off a form of severe neurological damage in infants that can lead to early death		
PHOSPHORUS	Helps build and protect bones and teeth. Part of DNA and RNA. Helps convert food into energy. Part of phospholipids, which carry lipids in blood and help shuttle nutrients into and out of cells	M: 700 mg, W: 700 mg	31-70: 4,000 mg 71+: 3,000 mg
POTASSIUM	Balances fluids in the body. Helps maintain steady heartbeat and send nerve impulses.	M: 4.7 g, W: 4.7 g	Not known

Needed for
muscle
contractions. A
diet rich in
potassium seems
to lower blood
pressure.
Getting enough
potassium from
your diet may
benefit bones

| SELENIUM | Acts as an antioxidant, neutralizing unstable molecules that can damage cells. Helps regulate thyroid hormone activity | M: 55 mcg, W: 55 mcg | 400 mcg |

| SODIUM | Balances fluids in the body. Helps send nerve impulses. Needed for muscle contractions. Impacts blood | M: 2,300 mg, W: 2,300 mg | Not determined |

	pressure; even modest reductions in salt consumption can lower blood pressure		
SULFUR	Helps form bridges that shape and stabilize some protein structures. Needed for healthy hair, skin, and nails	Unknown	Unknown
ZINC	Helps form many enzymes and proteins and create new cells. Frees vitamin A from storage in the liver. Needed for immune system, taste, smell, and wound healing. When taken with	M: 11 mg, W: 8 mg	40 mg

certain

antioxidants,

zinc may delay

the progression

of age-related

macular

degeneration

Proper balance and adequate levels of essential nutrients is important for a range of complex processes in our body. When vitamins are taken as supplements, they are introduced into the body at levels that could never be achieved by eating even the healthiest of diets. Supplementation can also result in large doses of a single vitamin being eaten 'alone.' When vitamins are consumed, they have many companions to help them along the way. For instance, vitamin A (beta-carotene) in food is accompanied by hundreds of its carotenoid relatives.

The RDA (Recommended Dietary Allowance) and the AI (Adequate Intake) are the amounts of a vitamin or mineral you need to keep healthy and stay well-nourished. They're tailored to women, men, and specific age groups. The UL (Tolerable Upper Intake Level) is the maximum number of daily vitamins and minerals that you can safely take without risk of an overdose or serious side effects. For certain nutrients, the higher you go above the UL, the greater the chance you'll have problems. Separate from the RDA and the UL, the Food and Drug Administration uses a different measure for the nutrients you need. The DV (Daily Value) is the only measurement you'll find on food and supplement labels. That's because space is limited, and there's a need for one single reference number. That number is the amount of a vitamin or nutrient that you should get for top health from a diet of 2,000 calories a day. The DV is sometimes the same as the RDA. Please consult with your primary doctor or healthcare professional prior to taking any multi-vitamin, herb, or supplement.

Vitamins	Recommended daily intake	Over dosage (mg or µg/d)
Biotin (B-complex)	30 µg	No information found
Folate (B-complex)	400 µg	Doses larger than 400 µg may cause anemia and may mask symptoms of a vitamin B_{12} deficiency
Vitamin A	600 µg	Extremely high doses (>9000 mg) can cause dry, scaly skin, fatigue, nausea, loss of appetite, bone and joint pains and headaches
Vitamin B_1 (thiamin)	1,4 mg	No toxic effects resulting from high doses have been observed

Vitamin B$_2$ (riboflavin)	1,6 mg	Doses higher than 200 mg may cause urine color alteration
Vitamin B$_3$ (niacin)	18 mg	Doses larger than 150 mg may cause problems ranging from facial flushing to liver disease
Vitamin B$_5$ (pantothenic acid)	6 mg	Dose should not exceed 1200 mg; this may cause nausea and heartburn
Vitamin B$_6$ (pyridoxine)	2 mg	Doses larger than 100 mg may cause numbness and tingling in hands and feet
Vitamin B$_{12}$ (cobalamin)	6 µg	Doses larger than 3000 µg may cause eye conditions
Vitamin C (ascorbic acid)	75 mg	No impacts of over dose have been proven so far

Vitamin D (cholecalciferol)	5 µg	Large doses (>50 µg) obtained from food can cause eating problems and ultimately disorientation, coma and death
Vitamin E (tocopherol)	10 mg	Doses larger than 1000 mg cause blood clotting, which results in increased likelihood of hemorrhage in some individuals
Vitamin K	80 µg	Large doses of one form of vitamin K (menadione or K_3) may result in liver damage or anemia
Minerals	Recommended daily intake	Over dosage
Boron	< 20 mg	No information found
Calcium	1000 mg	Doses larger than 1500 mg may cause stomach problems for sensitive individuals
Chlorine	3400 mg (in chloride form)	No information found

Chromium	120 µg	Doses larger than 200 µg are toxic and may cause concentration problems and fainting
Copper	2 mg	As little as 10 mg of copper can have a toxic effect
Fluorine	3,5 mg	No information found
Iodine	150 µg	No information found
Iron	15 mg	Doses larger than 20 mg may cause stomach upset, constipation, & blackened stools
Magnesium	350 mg	Doses larger than 400 mg may cause stomach problems and diarrhea
Manganese	5 mg	Excess manganese may hinder iron adsorption
Molybdenum	75 µg	Doses larger than 200 µg may cause kidney problems and copper deficiencies

Nickel	< 1 mg	Products containing nickel may cause skin rash in case of allergies
Phosphorus	1000 mg	Contradiction: the FDA states that doses larger than 250 mg may cause stomach problems for sensitive individuals
Potassium	3500 mg	Large doses may cause stomach upsets, intestinal problems or heart rhythm disorder
Selenium	35 µg	Doses larger than 200 µg can be toxic
Sodium	2400 mg	No information found
Vanadium	< 1,8 mg	No information found
Zinc	15 mg	Doses larger than 25 mg may cause anemia and copper deficiency

Some experts believe a vitamin's effectiveness can be altered by when and how a person consumes vitamins. Time of day, food, and liquid intake can have negative or positive effects on how well a vitamin works and how much of the vitamin is absorbed by the body. They argue that a vitamin cannot replace a healthy, well-rounded diet. B vitamins (thiamin, riboflavin, vitamin-B6, niacin, biotin, vitamin-B12, folic acid, and pantothenic acid) are used for energy boosts and stress reduction. Each of the 8 B vitamins have a separate function for the body. These B vitamins can be taken at the same time. In fact, companies offer vitamin complexes, which are combinations of the daily amount of each of the 8 B vitamin types. The best time of day to take a B vitamin is after waking up. Taking B vitamins on an empty stomach is supposed to help with absorption of the vitamin. Taking B vitamins also tend to increase energy, so taking them too late in the day may affect a person's ability to fall asleep.

Some experts believe the body absorbs and utilizes certain things best at certain times, in certain combinations, and in certain states. Some vitamins, minerals, and other supplements must be taken with food yet others require a fasted state for dedicated absorption; some are fat-soluble, meaning they can only be absorbed in the simultaneous presence of dietary fat (one of the many reasons fat intake is absolutely crucial!); some are water-soluble, meaning they do not require fat to be absorbed; some benefit from an insulin spike for full absorption; and still others must be spaced far from specific other supplements due to similar absorption pathways which hinder each other if conducted simultaneously.

Best times to take different types of vitamins:

1. Before breakfast:
    a.   Iron with citrus
    b.   Half dosage of B vitamins
    c.   Half dosage of calcium
2. During breakfast:
    a.   Half dosage of vitamin C
    b.   1 dosage of fish oil
3. Before lunch: half dosage of B vitamins
4. During lunch:

a.   Vitamin D with healthy fats

b.   Half dosage of vitamin C

c.   2nd dose of fish oil

5. During dinner: half dosage of calcium

6. Before or after meals: Probiotics can be taken prior to or following meals.

Some experts recommend you take your multi-vitamin, vitamin S, and any fat-soluble vitamin with a meal inclusive of healthy fats. Years ago, I heard a nurse recommend to take multivitamins and or supplements at night for optimal results due uninterrupted processing of these supplements by our bodies when we sleep.

Some supplements contain ingredients to help preserve their appearance and effectiveness.

1. Fillers: These are used to "bulk" a product up so that it's actually less potent than it looks. If a product in powder form is unusually inexpensive, you should take another look at the ingredient list for any fillers.

2. Binders: These are products that hold ingredients together, usually to keep them in the "shape" of a tablet. They may also be used to add volume if the amount of the active ingredient in the actual pill is very low. Lactose and sucrose are sometimes used as binders, so those who are lactose intolerant should pay careful attention.

3. Coatings: Coatings such as gelatin are sometimes used to make capsules smoother and easier to swallow. Gelatin is made from animal products, so vegans will want to look for other options.

4. Coloring and flavoring: Many inexpensive products like vitamins use artificial colors to make them look more appealing. In most cases these will be natural, but it's worth taking a look at the labels.

Finding a good multi-vitamin can be challenging. A lot of supplements claiming to be organic or all natural contain harmful synthetic preservatives. GMOs (Genetically Modified Organisms) can commonly be hidden in toxic vitamins and supplements, particularly Vitamin B12, B2, C and E. Key ingredients that signify GMO products in the vitamins include maltodextrin (from corn), ascorbic acid, as well as soy and rice proteins. If you are trying to avoid GMOs, then, you'll need to find vitamins and supplements that are USDA organic or Non-GMO Project Verified.

Toxic ingredients in supplements:

1. Artificial Food Coloring:

    Blue 2 Lake, FD&C Yellow No. 5 Lake, FD&C and Yellow No. 6 have been associated with a host of disturbing effects on the brain, central nervous system, and health of cells. All artificial food colorings approved by the FDA (Food & Drug Administration): FD&C Blue No. 1, FD&C Blue No. 2,   FD&C Green No. 3, FD&C Red No. 3, FD&C Red No. 40,   FD&C Yellow No. 5, and FD&C Yellow No. 6.

2. Sodium Benzoate:

    Consumers should be aware of anything containing benzene as it has been linked to various cancers. Sodium benzoate can form benzene if it's taken with ascorbic acid. Sodium benzoate has the potential to damage cells and DNA.

3. Hydrogenated Oils:

    Hydrogenated soybean oil is one of the major fillers in the majority of vitamins today. Unless soy is organic, it's probably genetically modified.

4. Lead, Mercury, & PCBs (polychlorinated biphenyls):
    Fish high on the food chain can accumulate mercury, lead, and other contaminants, those metals can make their way into your fish oil supplements. You don't want a toxic heavy metal or some PCBs with your

EFAs (essential fatty acids). Be careful of what brand of Omega-3 or EFAs you take. Make sure you carefully choose a brand that has been meticulously tested for lead or mercury contaminants. Your best choices should state that they are "Molecularly distilled and 3rd party tested to ensure PCBs, dioxins, mercury, lead and other contaminants are below acceptable limits set by the Council for Responsible Nutrition and other advisory agencies," or something similar.

5. Talc or Magnesium Silicate:

Magnesium Silicate is talc (as in talcum powder or baby powder) and it's used as an anti-caking agent in powder supplements. Studies have linked it to stomach cancer and lung inflammation. Talc is not currently considered food grade by the FDA. Although they were considering setting upper limits for asbestos fibers and adding it to the GRAS list way back in 1979.

6. Titanium Dioxide:

The International Agency for Research on Cancer has listed this ingredient as a possible carcinogen. Titanium dioxide has been shown to cause lung inflammation and damage, so it's yet another substance that has impact on workers at the production level. It has also been implicated in immune system function, with some studies showing DNA damage by Titanium dioxide nanoparticles, albeit marginal damage. Just a wee bit of DNA damage with your vitamins. Taken internally, it has been shown to cause kidney damage in mice and to induce small intestine inflammation. This is scary considering how many people suffering from Crohn's and gluten sensitivity are probably taking supplements containing Titanium dioxide.

7. Magnesium Stearate / Stearic Acid
8. Soy Lecithin and other hexane-extracted additives:

In addition to being made from GMO soy, this additive often contains solvents. The processing usually involves hexane. The processing done to remove the hexane can leave trace amounts. That residue is unregulated by the FDA even though it is listed by that organization as a potential carcinogen and neurotoxin — meaning there can still be hexane in your vitamins.

9. Mono- and Diglycerides:

These additives can contain trans fats.

10.   BHT:

This ingredient is believed to be a carcinogen. Butylated Hydroxytoluene is a preservative used in a range of products (including petroleum, cosmetics and even embalming fluid) to improve the shelf-life of fat-based products. It is an antioxidant which prevents the breakdown of fats. Though it's use is controversial, it has been linked to liver toxicity and some forms of cancer.

11.   Maltodextrin and ascorbic acid:

These common ingredients are made from GMO corn.

It's important to understand that supplements may contain additives from naturally-derived sources. Examples of common additives that are generally safe include stabilizers like xanthan gum and calcium sulphate, as well as calcium chloride and magnesium sulphate, which are sometimes used as firming agents. Antioxidant vitamins like A, C and E, as well as their derivatives (e.g.: citric acid) are also used as natural preservatives in supplements. Plant cellulose is an example of a filler that is often used as a binder or coating -- it is perfectly natural and safe.

Here are some things you can do:

1. Research ingredients that are banned in Europe, since they have stricter food regulation laws there.

2. Buy non-GMO, organic and vegan where possible or necessary.

3. Anything in a propyl or ethyl group is likely highly synthesized and should be avoided.

4. As a general rule of thumb, the less ingredients there are, the better it probably is.

5. Buy pure whenever possible – bulk powders, pure liquids and capsules (rather than tablets) are less likely to contain harmful ingredients.

6. Look for words that you recognize on the labels. Often times, for instance, rice flour or rice concentrate can be used is used instead of synthetic anti-caking agents or fillers.

7. Have a conversation! Any solid business – whether it's the supplier or the actual manufacturer – should be happy to answer your questions.

8. Be extra careful when buying "cheap" products online – if something is unusually inexpensive, it probably means it just has less of the actual substance in the package to begin with.

You may be wondering if you were to start taking vitamins or supplements today, how long will it take for you to see results. In other words, how long does it take for supplements to work?

Factors that determine length of time to see results:
1. Severity of Deficiency:
   The biggest factor that dictates how long before a supplement kicks in, is how deficient you are to begin with. Let's say nutrient stores are like pools. If your pool is empty, it's going to take longer to fill than if your pool is half or mostly full.
2. Supplement Dosage:
   The next factor is how much of the supplement you are taking. Going back to the pool, it's half full, but if you're only putting in a 5 gallon bucket each day, it's going to take a very long time to fill.

And that's not counting what the sun will evaporate and if you get sick of the pool never filling and give up. PLEASE REMEMBER NOT TO TAKE TOO MUCH OF ANY VITAMIN OR SUPPLEMENT.

3. Supplement Quality:

The quality of the supplement comes in next. In the US there is no federal regulation on supplements, meaning purchases of vitamins, minerals and herbs are completely unregulated by the US government, unless the supplement kills someone dead. All supplementation inspection of quality is optional and at the company's expense. Reputable companies will pay that. If you're trying to fill the pool with a hose that doesn't function, it's not going to fill.

4. Nutrients need other nutrients:

All nutrients need other nutrients for their absorption and utilization. For instance, magnesium is required in over 300 enzymatic processes. If you're supplementing with calcium, magnesium or zinc, yet deficient in vitamin D, you're not absorbing those minerals. If you're supplementing with iron, but deficient in vitamin A (beta-carotene), several B vitamins, vitamin C or zinc, you're having issues ranging from absorption to utilization.

5. Cause of Deficiency: What's causing the deficiency in the first place? Why is your pool empty in the first place? Is it a genetic situation? Is it a side effect of a medication? Do you need to make dietary changes? Have you been stressed and not realized that essentially drains your body of many nutrients, especially zinc? If you don't resolve what's draining the pool, you may never top it off with water, let alone keep it topped off.

6. **Food:**

Best for last: remember that supplement means "in addition to," not "in place of." The nutrients we need for health are the same ones we're intended to get from our food. If you don't know how to do so, don't feel dumb. Millions of Americans aren't sure of this. Speak with a nutrition professional to pair your supplemental efforts with a healthy diet. While you get the hang of a new way of eating, taking your supplements *in addition to* what you're eating will help fill in the gaps.

The bad news is that supplementation no longer sounds like an instant fix. It never was and never will be. Supplements are meant to be taken in addition to eating well and, in certain situations, to help those with medical conditions that affect nutrient status. Any supplement is going to take a minimum of 2 to 4 weeks to begin to work before person feels them 'kick in.' If it's a mineral, you're looking at about 90 days before your deficiency is fully amended because you're asking your body to absorb a rock. That said pairing your mineral supplement with healthy diet, you'll start to feel the difference in 2 to 4 weeks as well.

Most importantly, remember to consult with your primary doctor prior to taking any multi-vitamin, mineral, herb, or supplement.

Herbs are plants with savory or aromatic properties that are used for flavoring and garnishing food, medicinal purposes, or for fragrances; excluding vegetables and other plants consumed for macronutrients. Culinary use typically distinguishes herbs from spices. *Herbs* generally refers to the leafy green or flowering parts of a plant (either fresh or dried), while *spices* are usually dried and produced from other parts of the plant, including seeds, bark, roots and fruits. General usage of the term "herb" differs between culinary herbs and medicinal herbs.

Top herbs for your health:

(One 1 or more of the following herbs are available at herb-pharm.com.)

Sensory Perception:

Give your vision and hearing a boost by taking these herbs.

1. Ginkgo Biloba: Ginkgo has been attached to many potential benefits, but perhaps one of the most significant is its ability to improve blood flow to the eyes especially in those suffering from macular degeneration. It

can also be valuable to your ears as numerous studies have suggested it can help prevent tinnitus and inner ear disturbances as well as a number of other conditions.

2. Bilberry: A relatively unknown but powerful antioxidant, bilberry has a number of positive health effects for the brain and heart. It can also help to protect the retina and improve range and clarity of vision.

3. Passionflower: If staring at a computer screen or reading in dim light has your eyes strained, try taking a passionflower supplement. It can help relax the small blood vessels in the eye and make seeing easier.

4. Goldenseal: Sties and conjunctivitis can be irritating and embarrassing conditions. Take some goldenseal to help reduce the inflammation associated with these conditions and get you on the road to recovery.

5. Aspalathus: This South African herb contains a number of antioxidants that are similar to those found in Bilberry. These can boost your eye health while giving you overall improved immune function.

6. Mahonia Grape Extract: The sun can have an immensely damaging effect on the eyes, but this herb can help reduce the impact of sun damage while strengthening the retina, slowing eye aging and maintaining better overall eye health.

7. Bilwa: Found in the sub-Himalayan forests, this fruit has been used in India to help treat painful eye conditions like sties and conjunctivitis.

8. Mullein flower: This flowering plant can be a natural way to help rid yourself of an ear infection as it acts as a natural bactericide when condensed to oil form.

Mental Health and Function:

Keep your mind sharp, alert and in good health with a little help from these plants.

9. Kava kava: This herb can help calm your anxieties by binding to brain receptors that promote relaxation.

10.   St. John's Wort: Those with mild to moderate depression may find some relief with this herb. Numerous studies have been done on it, most finding that it can be as effective as some prescription drugs at treating depression. Those with more severe depression should, of course, consult a medical professional.

11.   Valerian: Lull your body into a restful sleep with a natural remedy instead of prescription pills. Valerian has been shown to be as effective as traditional sleeping pills, while eliminating some of the more harmful side effects associated with them.

12.   Bacopa: Used in India for several thousand years, this flowering plant has been said to improve memory, learning and cognition. Studies have shown that it can do little to improve your old memories but does have an effect on newly acquired information, so start taking it sooner rather than later.

13.   Ginseng: Many people have heard of the herb ginseng, but few know that there have been numerous studies done to document its effects. These studies seem to suggest that there can be some benefits of taking it that include improved memory and other mental performance and a whole host of other effects ranging from immune system stimulation to lowered cholesterol.

14.   Holy Basil: Also known as tulsi, this herb is not usually used in cooking like its cousin, but instead can help reduce the effects of stress on the body by inhibiting cortisol.

15.   Chamomile: Generally known as a relaxing herb, chamomile tea can be a great way to wind down after a stressful day and ease stress. Some also use it to calm nerves or relieve menstrual cramps.

16.   Suma: This rainforest plant can in some people help to normalize body systems and reduce the effects of stress.

17.   Brahmi: Give this Indian remedy a try to help boost your brain function and information retention.

18.   Gotu Kola: Commonly used in India, this herb can help to improve cognitive function and reduce anxiety, helping you think more clearly and calmly.

19.   Sage: Modern research has shown that sage can actually help make you wiser, improving memory and reducing inflammation.

20.   Kudzu: Feel like you'd like to have better self-control when it comes to drinking and killing all those brain cells? This herb can help you to curb your appetite for booze by helping alcohol more quickly get to the part of the brain that tells you enough is enough.

21.   Catnip: Not just for cats, this common herb when eaten can help reduce anxiety and produce an overall sedated effect.

Digestive and Urinary Systems:

Use these herbs to ensure that your plumbing stays in good condition.

22.   Licorice: You may love the taste of licorice but might not have known about the beneficial health effects it can have. It can soothe and relax gastrointestinal tissues, helping ease the pain of ulcers and acid reflux and has even been shown to help increase bile production.

23.   Milk Thistle: Give your liver some help filtering out all those toxins by taking some milk thistle. It can help improve the regeneration of liver tissue and regulate liver function as demonstrated in testing done at radiology tech schools nationwide.

24.   Peppermint Oil: A little dab of peppermint oil will do you to help relax the smooth muscles of your colon, stopping cramps and constipation that can be common symptoms of irritable bowel syndrome.

25.   Ginger: An upset stomach is never fun to deal with, but ginger may be the solution that you're looking for. Ginger helps slow the production

of serotonin, a major factor in the nauseated feeling you get when you are motion sick or experiencing pregnancy sickness.

26.   Senna: If you're feeling constipated, this herb may work well as a natural laxative to get things moving again.

27.   Gentian: This super bitter herb has been used for generations to treat digestive problems. Its bitter taste stimulates the digestive system, making it easier to get food through your system problem free.

28.   Uva Ursi: Try out this herb for a great natural way to help prevent getting bladder infections

29.   Aloe: While great for healing burns and skin irritation when applied topically, this plant can act as a helpful laxative when consumed.

30.   Gamma Orizanol: Give this remedy a try if you want to help calm an upset stomach.

31.   Rose Hips: These small berries serve a dual purpose helping to reduce bladder infections and to fight constipation.

32.   Agrimony: If your whole digestive system needs a lift, try out this herb, said to improve stomach, liver, kidney and gallbladder function.

33.   Anise: This licorice-flavored herb can help prevent the accumulation of painful gas in the stomach and intestines.

34.   Celery Seed: Those having a little difficulty urinating may want to try this natural remedy out, cited for its diuretic properties.

Physical Appearance:

Help yourself look good at any age with these powerful herbs.

35.   Burnet: The leaves of this plant have been used for thousands of years in China, and can help treat several skin conditions as well as reducing the inflammation of hemorrhoids and helping heal burns.

36.   Burdock: Used all over the world, this substance helps combat hair loss, treats dandruff, and helps skin problems.

37.   Calendula: Great for all around skin care, this herb can treat everything from acne to chapped lips.

38.   Comfrey: Use the leaves and roots of this plant to soothe skin irritations and promote connective cell growth.

39.   Plantain leaf: Because it has many soothing elements, this plant is one of the best remedies for cuts, skin infections, and chronic skin problems.

40.   Red Clover: If you've tried everything to get rid of your acne, why not give this natural acne and skin clearing remedy a try?

41.   Sassafras Leaf: Said to purify and cleanse the body, this plant can be a helpful tool in getting acne under control.

42.   Solomon's Seal Root: Make a wash out of this plant to help control skin problems and blemishes.

43.   Spikenard: Acne, pimples, blackheads, and rashes don't stand a chance against this inflammation fighting herb.

Heart and Circulatory System:

Give your heart and the blood throughout your body some healthy help with these herbs.

44.   Garlic: Garlic is a powerhouse when it comes to heart health. Regular usage has been shown to prevent cardiovascular disease and lower high blood pressure. In addition, studies suggest that it might help prevent cancer, kill bacteria, and even improve levels of t-cells in AIDS patients.

45.   Hawthorn: The berries of this flowering shrub are great for the heart, by helping to open up the coronary arteries, lowering blood

pressure, or slowing a rapid heart rate. Users will see the best effects after six months or more of taking the supplement.

46.   Guggul: Guggul is thought to bind to cholesterol in your gut so that you eliminate it before it enters your bloodstream, helping reduce your overall cholesterol and feel better.

47.   Horse chestnut: Help prevent those unsightly varicose veins by taking some horse chestnut. Aescin and other compounds in the herb can help bulk up weak capillaries and veins, making them less prone to swelling and pain.

48.   Cinnamon: If you're worried about the health of your circulatory system, consider adding a little cinnamon to your diet. Cinnamon has been shown to reduce blood sugar and help lower cholesterol.

49.   Dandelion: Dandelions are more than just an annoying weed; they can also be an effective way to help control high blood pressure. Researchers think it works like many prescription medicines, decreasing your blood volume and thereby your blood pressure.

50.   Angelica root: Traditional wisdom places this herb as a great heart strengthener, especially for those suffering from heart related conditions.

51.   Coriander: The seeds of the cilantro plant can help build and strengthen your circulatory system and make for a stronger, healthier heart.

52.   Cayenne: Containing capsicum, cayenne can help normalize blood pressure, increase the elasticity of blood vessels, and even slow bleeding.

53.   Motherwort: This plant has a long history of use and contains the alkaloid leonurine which can have a relaxing effect on smooth muscles like those found in the heart.

54.   Gynostemma: This herb has been shown in laboratory studies to have
a direct effect on the circulatory system, strengthening the heart and
helping wounds heal more quickly.

Pain and Inflammation:

Don't suffer through pain and inflammation, try these remedies instead.

55.   Arnica: The yellow flowers of this plant provide powerful anti-
inflammatory properties. Apply it to the skin to help reduce the pain
and swelling of bruises, strains and sprains.

56.   Feverfew: Several studies have confirmed that feverfew can help
prevent and treat migraines. It works by reducing the amount of serotonin
in the body and relaxing constricted blood vessels in the head.

57.   Willow Bark: A component of traditional aspirins, willow bark can
be a wonderful way to naturally reduce minor aches and pains.

58.   Devil's Claw: Native to southern Africa, this long-used remedy can
be a helpful agent in reducing inflammation as well as back and neck
pain.

59.   Chinese Skullcap: Part of the mint family, this herb can help
reduce stress headaches, the effects of PMS and even insomnia.

60.   Marjoram: Great for general aches and pains, this common herb can
be even more effective when combined with chamomile or gentian.

61.   Thyme: Many use thyme in their cooking without being aware that it
can help fight infection, reduce the pain of migraines and help clear
out the lungs.

62.   Meadowsweet: Meadowsweet contains many of the chemicals used to
make aspirin in its roots and when chewed can prove a helpful remedy for
headaches.

63.   Cat's Claw: While few definitive studies have been done, many
believe this herb can reduce general inflammation and boost the immune
system.

64.   Wood Betony: This attractive woodland plant does more than just
look pretty, it can also be used to reduce the pain associated with
headaches.

65.   Witch Hazel: Those suffering from hemorrhoids especially will
appreciate the anti-inflammatory properties of this herb.

Illness Prevention and Treatment:

Check out these herbs and plants to help keep you in general good health.

66.   Ephedra: One of the oldest cultivated medicinal herbs, Ephedra is
most commonly used to help treat and prevent colds. It works by dilating
the bronchial tubes through the release of adrenaline to be especially
useful to those suffering from allergies and asthma. Long term usage can
be harmful, however, so take it with care.

67.   Echinacea: Give your immune system a boost by taking some
echinacea. It activates the body's natural defense mechanism, white blood
cells, and helps your body prevent and fight off harmful infections and
bacteria.

68.   Astragalus: The Chinese have known about and used this herb for
thousands of years for a variety of different ailments. Recent studies
have shown that it may have a very real effect on the immune system,
increasing immune activity and effectiveness.

69.   Elderberry: Keep the flu at bay by chomping down on this berry.
Rich in vitamins A and C, it's been shown to prevent the flu virus from
spreading to healthy cells and cuts recovery time in half.

70.   Andrographis: Help keep your colds short and sweet by taking a
little bit of this herb. Studies have shown it can help reduce symptoms
like fatigue, sleeplessness, sore throat, and runny nose up to 90%.

71.   Kelp: Kelp is very high in iodine which is a natural infection fighter. As a bonus, it contains substances that are beneficial to hair and nails.

72.   Yarrow: While too much yarrow can be quite dangerous, a careful amount can be a great assistor in breaking a fever and fighting off a cold or flu.

73.   Boneset: An infusion of this herb can help you to more quickly fight off a cold.

74.   Elder: When you feel a cold or the flu coming on, enjoy some herbal tea made from this plant. If you are growing it at home, never eat the green parts of the plant as they are poisonous.

75.   Pleuresy root: Sometimes also called butterfly weed or Indian paintbrush, this variety of milkweed can help you get more out of your coughs when you have a cold or soothes some of the inflammation as well.

76.   Pau d'arco: This Brazilian herb is thought to be an all-around booster to your immune system.

77.   Maitake: Check out this mushroom, common in Asian medical practice for a jump start for your immune system as well as for help with blood pressure and cholesterol.

78.   Horehound: Sore throats and coughs can be remedied by making a tea of the leaves of this plant.

Diseases and Conditions:

While not cure-alls, these herbs and plants can help reduce the symptoms and severity of a variety of medical conditions.

79.   Khella: Check out this Middle Eastern herb for a little help on preventing those asthma attacks before they start. It dilates your bronchial tubes and relaxes the muscles that spasm during an attack, helping keep you breathing easy.

80.   Gymnema: Help reduce the effects of your diabetes symptoms by stimulating your pancreas to pump out more insulin with this herb. Used for thousands of years, recent preliminary studies have shown that it can have a big impact on reducing blood sugar.

81.   Eyebright: Don't let hay fever leave you knocked out with red eyes and a runny nose. This herb can help make your immune system less reactive to airborne allergens, making your life a little easier during allergy season.

82.   Lemon Balm: While there is no cure for herpes, there are ways that you can help make it a little more bearable, both in its genital and cold sore forms. Lemon balm can help reduce itching, swelling, and tingling while speeding up healing.

83.   Rosemary: While rosemary itself may not have any proven medical benefits, the application of it to other foods can. Studies have shown that rosemary helps prevent the formation of carcinogens caused by grilling foods.

84.   Wild Cherry: Wild cherry isn't just a soda flavoring; it can also help with asthma by loosening phlegm in the chest and throat and reduce inflammation of tissues.

85.   Fenugreek seed: Try this multipurpose remedy for help with allergies, coughs, headaches and sore throat.

86.   Forsythia: If you fear you may have picked up Lyme disease, this flowering scrub may offer you some help by providing antibacterial properties to weaken the disease.

87.   Boswellia: This herb relieves symptoms of both osteoarthritis and rheumatoid arthritis, and can even work well for those who reacted negatively to other natural treatments.

88.   Turmeric: Those suffering from painful joints due to arthritis may be well advised to add a little turmeric into their diets. This spice,

used in curry, contains curcumin, a powerful anti-inflammatory substance which can help reduce the pain and swelling.

89.   Yucca Root: Yucca root reduces inflammation of the joints, making it a valuable remedy for arthritis.

90.   Nettle: Extracts of this plant have been used to treat conditions like arthritis, anemia and hay fever.

Reproductive Health:

Ensure that your reproductive organs are in good health with these herbal remedies.

91.   Sea Buckthorn: Women suffering from vaginal dryness may find a natural cure in this remedy. It contains palmitoleic acid which helps hydrate mucus membranes and keeps skin moisturized.

92.   Black Cohosh: Make menopause easier by checking out this herb, used by some Native American groups. It contains plant estrogens which can help regulate and balance your rapidly changing hormones.

93.   Chaste Berry: The small, peppery-tasting berries of this plant can offer some help to women coming off birth control or those who just need a little assistance in regulating their hormones and menstrual cycles.

94.   Dandelion: If you suffer from a large amount of fluid retention around your time of the month, consider taking dandelion. It has natural diuretic properties that help eliminate excess fluids.

95.   Dong Quai: This plant has estrogenic properties making it a good choice for women who want to balance their hormones and ease common PMS symptoms. Be advised that it can take up to a year to see results from taking it.

96.   Raspberry Leaf: Pregnant women should check with their doctors before taking this herb, but it's generally considered safe and can help ease the painful process of labor.

97.   Saw Palmetto: Get some help keeping your prostate in good health
with this herb. It reduces the symptoms of an enlarged prostate, in some
cases as much as a prescription medication, though it may not work for
every man.

98.   Damiana Leaf: This multipurpose herb can help deal with sexual
dysfunction issues in both men and women as well as helping to reduce
hot flashes associated with menopause.

99.   Sarsaparilla: With effects similar to the male hormone
testosterone, this herb can be a great way to stimulate the sex drive
in both men and women.

100.   Beth Root: Some have seen balancing effects on the hormones with
this herbal tincture, leading to normalized menstrual bleeding, reduced
effects of menopause and easier pregnancy.

Chapter 7

No Microwave

Until recently, people began to scrutinize the microwave. Up until several years ago, no one questioned the damage done to food heated or prepared in a microwave. In 2013, I stopped using the microwave altogether. A former supervisor told me that the microwave changes the molecular structure of this food as it is heated. Those who are against the microwave believe: (1) the microwave zaps food nutrition, (2) the microwave destroy breast milk and vitamin B12, (3) the microwave creates carcinogens in food, (4) the microwave can adversely impact blood cells, and (5) the microwave can change your heart rate. They believe the primary reason the microwave damages food is due to possible radiation leakage as food is being heated. Some experts believe the microwave is the best cooking option for preserving nutrients in food. They argue nutrients and or minerals will be lost when food is heated. They argue that this loss of nutrients and or minerals is not only attributed to the microwave, but all forms of cooking.

Eliminating the microwave made me cook more often. It forced me to cook more. I even know to how to prepare food dishes for others utilizing conventional seasonings and spices without tasting them. I learned how to season meats and other dishes proportionately when cooking for others. (e.g. so much of this seasoning, a dash of this seasoning, etc.) I also know how to prepare organic dishes.

Chapter 8

Grocery Store

Where you shop for your groceries is important. Often times the selection the grocery store offers determine which products you purchase. This has a direct impact on your personal nutritional and also your health. If you are able to shop at a grocery store that offers organic and or natural products, you should do so as frequently as possible.

My favorite grocery stores are Whole Foods and Kroger. Whole Foods has the most extensive selection of natural and or organic products nationwide. You really should look closely at their shelves. They add new products to their product selection, which makes the shopping experience more interesting.

In Michigan, there are 8 Whole Food stores in Michigan. I have been to several of them. I am also appreciative of how friendly and willingness of their staff to assist their customers to the best of their ability at all times. I personally have never walked into any Whole Foods and not received less than outstanding customer service.

I am also appreciative of how organized Whole Foods is overall. If you go to different Whole Foods grocery stores in different cities, you are more likely to find the same or similar product selection with the exception of a few items. Most of their products are affordable. The warm foods selection or "buffet bar" section and the catered or prepared foods section is where the price markup really exists. If I am not mistaken, there is a set price per pound.

I have never been inside of a Trader Joes. So, I cannot comment on what they do or lack to offer. I also appreciate Kroger. A lot of their stores offer natural and organic sections to their customers.

Chapter 9

Gluten-Free, Soy-Free, and Reduced Fried Food

Gluten is a general name for the proteins found in wheat, rye, barley and triticale – a cross between wheat and rye. Gluten can be found in many types of foods, even ones that would not be expected.

Wheat, Barley, and Rye:

Wheat is commonly found in:

1. Breads

2. Baked goods

3. Soups

4. Pasta

5. Cereals

6. Sauces

7. Salad dressings

8. Roux

Barley is commonly found in:

1. malt (malted barley flour, malted milk and milkshakes, malt extract, malt syrup, malt flavoring, malt vinegar)

2. food coloring

3. soups

4. beer

5. Brewer's Yeast

Rye is commonly found in:

1.   Rye bread, such as pumpernickel

2.   Rye beer

3.   Cereals

Triticale is a newer grain, specifically grown to be similar to wheat, while being tolerant to a variety of growing conditions like rye. It can potentially be found in:

1.   Breads

2.   Pasta

3.   Cereals

Gluten is found in many foods you may not be aware of, as well, such as:

1.   Potato chips

2.   Processed meats

3.   Flavorings

4.   Natural juices

Always read labels. If something is fried or coated, crispy or crusted, that could indicate that it was coated with breading or gluten-containing flour.

Gluten can also be found in non-food products:

1.   Shampoo

2.   Toothpaste

3.   Makeup

4.   Laundry detergent

5.   Mouthwash

Oats can add diversity and offer many nutritional benefits to the gluten-free diet. Celiac Disease Foundation's medical experts recommend only oats labeled gluten-free as cross-contact may occur when oats are grown side-by-side with wheat, barley or rye. Patients eating oats from any source may complain of symptoms. This could be due to one or more of several factors, including intolerance to the increase in fiber, food intolerances, contamination with gluten, or, rarely, the development of an immune response to oat protein, similar to that occurring due to gluten. The decision to include oats in your diet should be made with your physician or dietitian and should include monitoring of your anti-tissue transglutaminase (anti-tTG) antibody levels.

There are several types of proteins that make up the total protein content in cereal crops, one of which is gluten. Gluten is a protein composite that accounts for 75 to 85% of the total protein content in bread wheat. Gluten component proteins are found in the endosperm of mature wheat grain, where they form a continuous framework around the starch granules. Gluten is comprised of two protein groups: glutenin and gliadin. Glutenin contributes to the elastic character of gluten while gliadin contributes to extensibility. Gluten forms when water is added to flour and is mixed. During mixing, a continuous network of protein forms, giving the dough its strength and elasticity. By holding gas produced during fermentation, the protein network allows bread to rise. It also allows the dough to maintain its shape. These two functions of the protein network are what give bread its chewy texture.

Gluten is a water-insoluble protein that is formed when water is mixed with wheat flour. Proteins are very large molecules composed of amino acids. Two of the naturally occurring proteins in flour are called glutenin and gliadin. When sufficient water is added to dry flour the two proteins emerge. The process of wetting the proteins is called hydration. As water and flour are mixed the hydrated proteins are brought together and begin to interact. They literally begin to stick to each other through the formation of chemical bonds. These new chemical bonds are called cross-links. In the case of gluten, a number of different types of chemical bonds form between the proteins, with some (disulfide bonds) being stronger than others (ionic bonds and hydrogen bonds). Continued mixing causes more cross-links to form between the proteins until a large network of chemically linked proteins is formed. When dough is mixed or kneaded the hydrated flexible proteins are stretched and aligned in the direction of kneading providing more opportunities to form cross-links between the proteins. Kneading also incorporates air, which helps to form strong disulfide bonds. As kneading continues the protein networks combine to form sheets of proteins. The chemical cross-linking of glutenin and gliadin forms gluten, a very elastic substance.

Gluten is a controversial subject. Awareness of the negative health effects of gluten has increased in the past few years. One 2013 survey shows that a third of Americans are actively trying to eliminate gluten from their diets. Some experts believe gluten is harmless, while others believe gluten is harmful. Some believe there are health benefits associated with consumption of gluten. Some experts believe people are unnecessarily eliminating gluten from their diet if they have not been diagnosed with Celiac Disease and are not eating gluten. Some experts believe birth defects (primarily autism) can be attributed to consumption of gluten. Some experts believe gluten adversely impacts gut or gastrointestinal health.

An allergic reaction to gluten is celiac disease. The allergy is linked to an excessive immune response to partially digested gliadin. When gluten reaches the digestive tract and is exposed to the cells of the immune system, they mistakenly believe that it is coming from some sort of foreign invader, like a bacteria. In certain people who are sensitive to gluten, this causes the immune system to mount an attack against it. In celiac disease (the most severe form of gluten sensitivity), the immune system attacks the gluten proteins, but it also attacks an enzyme in the cells of the digestive tract called tissue transglutaminase. Therefore, gluten exposure in celiacs causes the immune system to attack both the gluten as well as the intestinal wall itself. For this reason, celiac disease is classified as an autoimmune disease. The immune reaction can cause degeneration of the intestinal wall, which leads to nutrient deficiencies, various digestive issues, anemia, fatigue, failure to thrive as well as an increased risk of many serious diseases.

Celiac disease is on the rise and most people remain undiagnosed. Celiac disease is believed to afflict about 1% of people, but it may be more common (over 2%) in the elderly. There are also studies showing that the rate of celiac disease is increasing rapidly in the population. Keep in mind that a large percentage of celiacs don't even have abdominal symptoms, making diagnosis on clinical grounds very difficult. The symptoms might manifest themselves in different ways, like fatigue, anemia... or something much worse, like a doubled risk of death in several studies. According to one study, over 80% of people with celiac disease don't even know that they have it. There are two sources showing that up to 6-8% of people may have gluten sensitivity, based on anti-gliadin antibodies found in the blood. However, one gastroenterologist found that 11% of people had antibodies against gluten in their blood and 29% of people had antibodies against it in stool samples. About 40% of people carry the HLA-DQ2 and HLA-DQ8 genes, which make people susceptible to gluten sensitivity.

Eighteen million Americans have a gluten sensitivity. Three million Americans have Celiac disease. Gluten sensitivity is a condition that causes a person to react after ingesting gluten. Symptoms include digestive issues such as gas, bloating, diarrhea and constipation, as well as fatigue, brain fog, joint and muscle aches, depression, anxiety, skin problems, migraines, dental issues, hormone imbalance and weight gain. Celiac disease is a genetic autoimmune disorder where eating gluten damages the small intestine. The nutrients cannot be absorbed properly into the body and it causes malnourishment. Symptoms include fatigue, anemia, bone and joint pain, arthritis, osteoporosis, depression, anxiety, tingling or numbness in hands and feet, seizures, migraines, missed periods, infertility, itchy skin rash, liver and biliary tract disorders, and canker sores in the mouth. It can even lead to the start of neurological diseases, or certain cancers. For people with celiac disease, a gluten-free diet is a must.

Some medical experts believe gluten is bad for your brain. Some medical experts believe gluten can influence behavior and mood, and can cause euphoria, addictive behavior and appetite stimulation. For some people, wheat affects them like a drug because it can yield drug-like neurological effects. The relationship of celiac disease to neurologic and psychiatric complications has been observed for over 40 years. Gluten sensitive patients also experience these complications. Data suggests that up to 22% of patients with celiac disease develop neurologic or psychiatric dysfunction, and as many as 57% of people with neurological dysfunction of unknown origin test positive for anti-gliadin antibodies (a sign of celiac disease). The research study Neurologic and Psychiatric Manifestations of Celiac Disease and Gluten Sensitivity sheds light onto just how damaging gluten can be to our brain.

Here are 7 neurological conditions that can be caused by gluten:

1. Ataxia: The best-characterized neurologic complication related to gluten sensitivity is ataxia, a lack of muscle control or coordination of voluntary movements, such as walking or picking up objects. Ataxia can affect various movements, creating difficulties with speech, eye movement and swallowing.

2. Epilepsy: Epilepsy is also affected by gluten sensitivity or celiac disease. Seizure activity was better managed in the patients who received the earliest gluten-free diets. A smaller study of four patients reported that three of the four patients had significant reduction of their seizure activity after going on a gluten-free diet. In another study of patients with epilepsy, of 7 patients diagnosed with celiac disease, after five months of going on a gluten-free diet, seizures were completely under control in 6 patients and antiepileptic drugs were discontinued.

3. Anxiety Disorders: Various types of anxiety are associated with gluten intolerance. One study found that celiac disease patients were significantly more likely to have anxiety when compared to controls, and that after one year on a gluten-free diet, there was a significant improvement in anxiety symptoms. Other anxiety disorders such as social phobia and panic disorder have been linked to gluten. It was reported that a significantly higher proportion of celiac disease patients had social phobia compared to normal controls. Additionally, a higher lifetime prevalence of panic disorder has been found in celiac disease patients with new studies confirming the increased association between celiac disease and anxiety.

4. Depression and Mood Disorders: Depression and related mood disorders are reported to be associated with gluten sensitivity and celiac disease. One study found that major depressive disorder and dysthymic disorder (a continuous long-term, chronic form of depression) were more common in a group of celiac disease patients compared to controls. Another study found that celiac patients were more likely to be diagnosed with subsequent depression as compared to people without the disease. Research found that an elderly population with gluten sensitivity was more than twice as likely to have depression when compared to the elderly sample without gluten sensitivity. Research has described improvement in depressive symptoms following a gluten-free diet. Research showed that short-term exposure to gluten specifically induced feelings of depression. This may explain why people with a gluten sensitivity feel better on a gluten-free diet.

5. Attention Deficit-Hyperactivity Disorder (ADHD): A few studies have suggested that ADHD may be associated with gluten intolerance, as well. A study measured ADHD symptoms in celiac disease patients and found that these symptoms are more common in them as compared to the general population. A six-month gluten-free diet was reported to improve ADHD symptoms and the majority of patients (74%) in this report wanted to continue the gluten-free diet due to significant relief of their symptoms. Research demonstrated that a gluten-free diet significantly improved ADHD symptoms in patients with celiac disease, suggesting that celiac disease should be included in the ADHD symptom checklist. After the initiation of the gluten-free diet, patients reported significant improvement in their behavior and functioning compared to the period before treatment.

6. Autism Spectrum Disorders: Autism spectrum disorders (ASD) have been associated with gluten intolerance. Studies have shown the relationship between ASD and autoimmune disease, specifically celiac disease. One study found an increased risk of ASDs in children with a maternal history of rheumatoid arthritis and celiac disease. When compared to controls, persons with ASDs and their family members have been found to have leaky gut syndrome, and when treated with a gluten- and casein-free diet, have been able to improve

leaky gut when compared to patients on an unrestricted diet. This has been supported by other studies.

7. Schizophrenia: Schizophrenia may be the psychiatric disorder with the most robust relationship to gluten. As early as 1953, it was noted that children with schizophrenia were prone to having celiac disease. A research study published in 1966 showed that the prevalence of schizophrenia was lower in areas of lower grain consumption. It also showed that a milk- and cereal-free diet improved schizophrenic symptoms. A similar study showed that these patients were discharged twice as quickly as those not on the diet and a third showed that recovery is disturbed when gluten is added to a previously gluten-free diet. Wheat protein was shown to cause reactions such as seizures and other unusual behaviors, and this may be related to the development of schizophrenia.

8. Other Neurological Disorders: Other neurological displays of gluten sensitivity and celiac disease include peripheral neuropathy (damaged nerves), inflammatory myopathies (muscle disease), myelopathies (disease of spinal cord), headache, and gluten encephalopathy (abnormal brain function). White matter abnormalities associated with gluten sensitivity have also been reported.

9. Hormone Decline Can Also Affect Your Brain: Did you know that hormone decline and imbalance can also cause symptoms such as brain fog, depression, moodiness and anxiety, to name a few?

Wheat is a grain. The calories in wheat come mostly from carbohydrates, but wheat also contains a few problem proteins.

1.   Gluten

2.   Wheat Germ Agglutinin

3.   Amylase Trypsin Inhibitors

Problems caused by these proteins are not the same thing as blood sugar problems caused by the carbohydrates in wheat. It's true that getting a majority of calories from wheat (especially refined wheat) can cause metabolic problems like blood sugar swings. But these problems would be caused by any high-carb diet, and they're only relevant for people eating a *large amount of wheat*: something like a spoonful of soy sauce wouldn't be a problem. This post is not about metabolic issues like blood sugar and carbohydrates. It's about a totally different list of problems caused specifically by wheat and the proteins it contains. These problems are relevant even for people eating a small amount of wheat, and even for people who do fine eating carbs.

Ways gluten and wheat can damage your health:

1. Wheat Problems Aren't Restricted to People with Celiac Disease:

The most famous problem with wheat is celiac disease, an autoimmune reaction provoked by gluten and treatable with a gluten-free diet. 30-40% of people have the genetic background to potentially develop celiac disease, but only about 1-3% of people actually do - it's not clear why but it may have something to do with the gut microbiome. Most people know that celiac disease requires absolutely strict avoidance of all gluten. But a lot of people also think that if you *don't* have celiac disease, you're completely in the clear. Some experts believe this is not true. Recently there's been an increased amount of interest in non-celiac gluten sensitivity (NCGS). Plenty of people have documented sensitivities to gluten that aren't actually celiac disease (as you'll read below, there's a different immune reaction involved). There's also the overlapping problem of other proteins in wheat - wheat germ agglutinin and amylase trypsin inhibitors are not the same thing as gluten and you can be sensitive to them regardless of how your body handles gluten.

2. Gut Inflammation:

Inflammation is the natural response of your immune system to injury. You can see it in action whenever you get a cut or splinter and the surrounding area gets all red and tender. The proteins in wheat are gut irritants: they're like that papercut or splinter digging into the lining of your gut, causing an inflammatory response. The most famous case is the inflammation caused by gluten in people with celiac disease or non-celiac gluten sensitivity. But inflammation from wheat is also a problem even for people who aren't sensitive to gluten specifically. Amylase trypsin inhibitors (ATIs for short) that can provoke an inflammatory immune response in the GI tract by stimulating immune cells. This occurs in people regardless of whether they have celiac disease or not - it's a completely different problem from gluten and it can cause trouble for you regardless of whether or not you're sensitive to gluten in particular.

3. Increased Intestinal Permeability:

Inflammation in the gut contributes to a problem called intestinal permeability. The gut has a very complex system of "border control" that lets digested food into your bloodstream (this is how you get nutrients from it) while keeping everything else out. Every day, you swallow millions of random viruses, bacteria, indigestible molecules like dust, and other stuff that needs to go out the other end, not into your bloodstream. Inflammation in the gut messes up that system of border control. It loosens the junctions between cells in the gut wall so too much stuff can pass through. This is often described as making the gut "leaky" (hence the popular name of "leaky gut"). On top of inflammation leading to increased permeability, gluten accelerates this process by stimulating the release of a protein called zonulin. Zonulin independently contributes to loosening the junctions between cells in the gut. Add together the inflammation and the zonulin, and wheat has a powerful effect on gut permeability, which is really a problem. Intestinal permeability is a big problem - most notably because it's an essential factor in the development of autoimmune diseases. There are also studies showing that individuals with neither celiac disease nor diagnosed gluten sensitivity have adverse reactions to gluten. In one of these studies, individuals with irritable bowel syndrome were randomized to either a gluten-containing or a gluten-free diet. The group on the gluten-containing diet had more pain, bloating, stool inconsistency and fatigue compared to the other group. There are also studies showing that gluten can cause inflammation in the intestine and a degenerated intestinal lining. Gluten may also have negative effects on the barrier function of the intestine, allowing unwanted substances to "leak" through into the bloodstream. However, according to one study, this "leakiness" of the gut only happens in celiac patients. Irritable bowel syndrome (IBS) involves various digestive issues with an unknown cause, afflicting about 14% of people in the U.S. According to the studies above, some cases of IBS may be either caused or exacerbated by gluten.

4. Double Trouble: Wheat Germ Agglutinin:

Wheat germ agglutinin is an inflammatory, immune-disrupting protein found in wheat and despite the similar name it isn't the same thing as gluten. Wheat germ agglutinin can provoke an inflammatory response in gut cells and disturb the natural immune barrier in the gut, making the gut more permeable to things that don't belong in your blood. Again, this is totally separate from the problem of gluten. Obviously, gluten and WGA usually come as a package deal, because they're both found in wheat, but you can have trouble with WGA even if you had no reaction to a gluten elimination challenge.

5. Increased Vulnerability to Gut Autoimmunity:

Items #1-4 on this list discussed how wheat makes the gut more permeable, so all kinds of stuff can get into the bloodstream even though it shouldn't be there. Included in that stuff is…gluten! Specifically, gliadin, which is a component of gluten. Once it's inside your bloodstream, gliadin runs into your immune system, and that's where the problems really start, in the form of molecular mimicry. Molecular mimicry works like this: some foreign thing gets into the bloodstream. The immune system forms antibodies against it. So far, so good: that's how the immune system is supposed to work. But if that foreign thing looks enough like your own body's tissue, then the antibodies formed to fight it might start attacking your own body as well. Molecular mimicry may be the reason why people with celiac disease mount an attack on their own gut cells: to your immune system, gliadin looks a lot like the cells lining the gut. But it's not just celiac disease! Gluten-related inflammation may also be a factor in the development of

Crohn's Disease, another autoimmune gut disease. In this study of patients with inflammatory bowel disease (Crohn's Disease and ulcerative colitis), a gluten-free diet helped a majority of people who tried it. And gut cells aren't the only cells affected by gluten-related autoimmunity.

6. Increased Vulnerability to non-Celiac Autoimmune Diseases:

There are a lot of studies linking gluten to all kinds of other autoimmune diseases, including autoimmune thyroid disorders, type 1 diabetes, fibromyalgia (for both celiac disease and non-celiac gluten sensitivity!), rheumatoid arthritis, autoimmune liver disease, and a couple different autoimmune skin diseases. The common factor here might be the gluten. Wheat gluten is a major potential trigger of Type 1 Diabetes (that's the autoimmune type, not the diet-and-lifestyle type). In this study, feeding mice a gluten-free diet reduced the rate of Type 1 diabetes in their children. There's also evidence that breastfeeding human children reduces the rate of type 1 diabetes, which would make sense if gluten is the problem because breastfeeding delays the introduction of gluten to the baby.

7. Autoimmune Reactions in People Without Celiac Disease:

Point #6 above gave a lot of reasons why celiac disease is associated with other autoimmune diseases, but it's not limited to people with celiac disease. If you thought non-celiac gluten sensitivity was unrelated to autoimmune disease, you thought wrong! This study found that a lot of people with non-celiac gluten sensitivity have autoimmune markers in their blood, suggesting that the wheat exposure might be causing autoimmune issues even without celiac disease. One interesting aspect of this is that patients with non-celiac gluten sensitivity may have a different type of autoimmune reaction, which just underlines that celiac disease and non-celiac gluten sensitivity are two different things. But the point is that both involve potentially serious autoimmune responses.

8. Damage to the Gut Biome:

Not the all-important gut biome! The gut biome, aka the gut microbiome, also known as the gut flora, is the collection of friendly bacteria that live in your gut. They help regulate your immune system, control intestinal permeability, digest your food, synthesize nutrients like vitamin K2, send hunger/fullness signals to your brain, and do all kinds of other stuff. People with celiac disease often have very bad problems with the gut flora, but those problems are significantly reduced when the person eliminates gluten. Once again, it's not limited to celiac disease: non-celiac gluten sensitivity also involves disturbances in the gut flora. Even in people who aren't sensitive to gluten at all, inflammation caused by other components of wheat can also rebound on the gut biome. And independently of any of that, wheat is also high in FODMAPs, which may be an issue for people with sensitivities to that.

9. Gastrointestinal Symptoms (Even for People who Don't have Celiac Disease):

Some experts believe gluten impacts gut bacteria and intestinal permeability, which has actual, noticeable consequences. Most of the direct damage involves the gut, so it makes sense to start there:

   a. In people with celiac disease, gluten causes immediate and severe symptoms (diarrhea and/or constipation, heartburn, pain, bloating, gas, stools that smell awful, sometimes vomiting).

   b. In people with non-celiac gluten sensitivity, symptoms are typically similar to celiac disease.

   c. Even in people who aren't sensitive to gluten specifically, the inflammatory action of other components of wheat (wheat germ agglutinin and amylase trypsin inhibitors) contributes to chronic, relapsing gut problems.

   Of course, there are non-wheat-related reasons why a person might have GI problems (stress is a biggie, and stress is certifiably gluten-free). But gluten can contribute to the problem, even if it's "only" a low-level inflammatory response that you've gotten used to. Sure, constipation and feeling bloated after meals might be your "normal," but what if it didn't have to be?

10.   Brain Symptoms:

Brain fog and fatigue are symptoms of both celiac disease and non-celiac gluten sensitivity. On a more serious note, the gut inflammation and microbiome disturbances involved in the immune-inflammatory response to gluten may increase vulnerability to dementia and Alzheimer's disease. Autoimmunity in general (whether it's celiac disease or some other gluten-related autoimmunity) may be involved in depression. This doesn't mean that gluten is the cause of all mental health problems or that eliminating gluten will cure them. Nobody is saying that. Mental health is complicated and there are all kinds of factors to consider. The point is that in some people, gluten may be one of them.

11.   Skin Symptoms:

The most famous cause of gluten-related skin problems is celiac disease, which can cause a skin disease called dermatitis herpetiformis. Symptoms of dermatitis herpetiformis include an itchy, red rash with raised blisters. Symptoms typically show up in a person's 20's. This isn't limited to celiac disease. This study describes the way non-celiac gluten sensitivity can show up as skin problems: "very itchy…similar to eczema, psoriasis, or dermatitis herpetiformis." The itchy skin showed up most often on the arms and legs. The upshot: wheat is pretty bad news even for people who don't have celiac disease. And the symptoms don't necessarily show up as dramatic episodes of vomiting and diarrhea. Try giving up gluten for a few weeks just to see how your body reacts.

A lot of products contain gluten-free labels. Most of these products contains rice ingredients as a gluten substitute. Studies have found alarming levels of arsenic in rice. Most of the rice today, whether white, brown, wild, organic, or conventional, is tainted with arsenic — one of the world's most toxic poisons.

Arsenic is naturally present in the environment. This mineral occurs in the Earth's crust and is found in soil, water, plants, and animals. Humans have complicated this issue by adding more arsenic to the soil through pesticides and fertilizers.

Arsenic exists in two forms: organic and inorganic. In this usage, organic does not refer to a type of farming. It's a chemistry term.

Arsenic combined with carbon is organic and mainly found in plant and animal tissues. Organic arsenic is utilized in pesticides and weed killers. Organic arsenic may be considered poisonous in high concentrations. Some experts believe organic arsenic can be linked to an increased risk of cancer. Organic arsenic is bound to carbon and hydrogen.

On the other hand, arsenic with no carbon (and combined with other elements) is inorganic and mainly found in rocks, soil, or water. The toxicity of arsenic varies widely. Both are considered public health concerns. Inorganic arsenic is generally considered more toxic than organic arsenic. Inorganic arsenic is most often used in pesticides and fertilizers. It's also found in a variety of foods. Chickens are often fed arsenic-containing drugs to make them grow faster. One of the most common food sources of inorganic arsenic is rice. Since rice is grown in flooded fields, it absorbs more arsenic from the environment than other crops. Rice and rice flour are the most common ingredients in gluten-free products and are often consumed multiple times a day.

You can't tell if arsenic is in your food or drinks because both organic and inorganic arsenic have no smell or taste. Most of the organic and inorganic arsenic you ingest will leave your body in a few days. But some of the inorganic arsenic — the kind of more concern — will remain in your body for months or even longer. Frequent exposure to inorganic arsenic, even in low doses, can cause health concerns.

Small doses of arsenic can cause:

1. Stomach aches

2. Headaches

3. Drowsiness

4. Abdominal pain and diarrhea

5. And confusion

Larger doses of arsenic create more serious problems. Inorganic arsenic can even be deadly. A dose the size of a pea was found to be fatal.

Long-term exposure to arsenic has been linked to numerous health issues, including:

1. Skin pigmentation and lesions

2. Dementia

3. Type 2 diabetes

4. High blood pressure and heart disease

5. Neurological problems

6. And other ailments

Arsenic is also a known human carcinogen. Arsenic is linked to many types of cancer, including skin, lung, bladder, liver, and kidney cancers. Evidence suggests lung cancer is the most common cause of arsenic-related mortality. The International Agency for Research on Cancer classified arsenic as a category 1 carcinogen, meaning it's *known to cause cancer in humans*. The U.S. EPA has also determined that inorganic arsenic is carcinogenic to humans. Inorganic arsenic is generally considered more harmful, but the IARC considers two types of organic arsenic to be "possibly carcinogenic to humans."

Arsenic is a concern for pregnant women and children. Pregnant women who are exposed to arsenic may put their unborn babies at risk of having compromised immune systems while in the womb and in early life. The

U.S. Food and Drug Administration found that high levels of inorganic arsenic during pregnancy are linked to numerous adverse outcomes. For example, exposure to arsenic during pregnancy and infancy can impair a child's performance on developmental tests.

Consumer Reports tested 223 samples of rice products and found significant levels of arsenic in almost all of them, including white, brown, parboiled, jasmine, basmati, and other types of rice. Arsenic was found in rice whether it was organic or conventional — and from all regions of the world. Brown rice is generally healthier than white rice. White rice is believed to be stripped of its outer layers, fiber, and beneficial nutrients. Consumer Reports found brown rice had 80% more arsenic than white rice. Some experts believe arsenic, along with other valuable nutrients, tends to collect in rice's brown outer hull. Black rice (also known as forbidden rice) is an ancient grain that has been found to have as many antioxidants as blueberries, but it will likely have higher levels of arsenic than white rice. Wild rice (technically not a rice but still a grain) may contain less arsenic, but it depends on the water where it grows. Organically-farmed rice may contain fewer pesticides, but all rice soaks up arsenic from the soil. So organic rice will have fewer toxins overall. But it won't likely have lower levels of arsenic unless the soil it grew in was never exposed to arsenic.

Basmati rice from California, India, or Pakistan is the best choice, according to Consumer Reports data. These types of rice have about one third of the inorganic arsenic compared to brown rice from other regions. Rice grown in Arkansas, Texas, Louisiana, and most other U.S. states had the highest inorganic arsenic levels. So, it's best to minimize or avoid rice grown in these areas. You can also check company websites and contact rice companies to see if they conduct independent testing for arsenic levels in their rice.

Arsenic-based pesticides were heavily used on crops for decades. And inorganic arsenic can persist in the soil indefinitely. Even if farmland has been growing organic food for decades, if it was *ever* exposed to arsenic-contaminated pesticides, these toxins may still persist in the soil today. Inorganic arsenic compounds and most arsenic-based pesticides have now been banned in agriculture in the U.S. But some may still reach Americans by way of other countries.

To some extent, arsenic can be washed off. Arsenic is water soluble. Published studies indicate that cooking rice in excess water (from six to 10 parts water to one-part rice), and draining the excess water, can reduce 40 to 60% of the inorganic arsenic content, depending on the type of rice. And a 2015 study published in PLOS ONE, found a cooking method that reduced arsenic by 85%. They used a filter coffee maker to pass the hot water through the rice as it cooked.

In my personal opinion, you should minimize your consumption of products containing rice ingredients. However, if you must have rice, you must take some precautions prior to consuming rice.

If you decide to eat rice, you may want to take these steps:

1. Choose organic basmati rice from California (or India and Pakistan) if possible.

2. Rinse rice thoroughly or even better soak it for 48 hours before cooking it, pouring off the water and rinsing it every 8 to 12 hours (like soaking beans).

3. Cook rice in 6 to 10 parts water to one-part rice.

4. When the rice is done, drain off the extra water after cooking.

Water is often contaminated with arsenic as well, so using filtered water is best.

The FDA issued a statement discouraging parents to not use rice and rice cereals as a primary food due to arsenic contamination. Instead, the agency advises parents to feed kids a variety of other foods.

High levels of inorganic arsenic have been found in many rice products.

For example:

1.   Rice milk

2.   Brown rice syrup

3.   Rice-based pasta

4.   Bread made with rice

5.   Cereals made with rice

6.   Crackers made with rice

7.   Cereal bars with rice or brown rice syrup

So, it's important to consider reducing the amount of all rice products you're eating. According to tests by Consumer Reports, only one serving of rice cereal or rice pasta could put kids over the maximum amount of rice they recommend in a week. And rice cakes give kids close to a weekly limit in only one serving!

If you are concerned about whether you are consuming a high level of arsenic, you may want to ask your primary doctor about testing.

There are several ways to test for arsenic in the body:

1. Arsenic 24-hour urine test: This is a preferred screening test. If this is elevated, it is necessary to differentiate between inorganic and organic arsenic. Inorganic is considered to be much more toxic.
2. Rapid urine spot test: This is not as accurate as the 24-hour urine test and does not differentiate between the two forms or arsenic: organic and inorganic.
3. Blood Test: May be utilized in conjunction with the 24-hour urine test to detect acute and recent arsenic exposure. It is also utilized to monitor levels.

The Food and Drug Administration (FDA) does not have standards for levels of arsenic in food. The EPA guideline for arsenic in water is 10 ppb, including bottled water. Consumer advocates are calling for the FDA to act quickly to regulate arsenic in rice.

I remember when soy was first introduced to the market. Soy was considered the best thing since sliced bread. The vegetarian and the vegan could have the best of both worlds.

Yet soy is controversial. Some experts believe soy is healthy. Some experts believe soy should be consumed in moderation but does offer health benefits. Some experts vilify soy. These experts believe soy should never be consumed. Some experts attribute infertility and birth defects to either moderate or excessive consumption of soy.

Soybeans and soy foods contain a variety of bioactive components, including saponins, protease inhibitors, phytic acid, and isoflavones. Isoflavones belong to a class of compounds generally known as phytoestrogens, plant compounds that have estrogen-like structures. The dominant isoflavone in soy is genistein, with daidzein and glycitein composing the remainder. Within soy, isoflavones are almost entirely bound to sugars, producing the respective compounds genistin, daidzin, and glycitin. Soy isoflavones have been linked with numerous health effects, but the strength of the relationships and whether the effects are beneficial are strongly debated. Soy isoflavones are frequently referred to as weak estrogens, and depending upon the specific circumstance, they can act as agonists, partial agonists, or antagonists to endogenous estrogens (such as estradiol) and xenoestrogens (including phytoestrogens) at estrogen receptors. They are not especially potent, however, and activity varies by tissue concentration, cell type, hormone receptor type, and stage of differentiation. In addition to their estrogen receptor activity, some experts believe soy isoflavones may also interfere with steroid metabolism by inhibiting aromatase, hydroxysteroid dehydrogenase, and steroid α-reductase, and by altering the ratio of estradiol metabolites. Soy isoflavones may also act as antioxidants; inhibitors of proteases, tyrosine kinases, and topoisomerases; inducers of Phase I and/or Phase II enzymes such as cytochrome P450s, glutathione *S*-transferase, and quinone reductase; and inhibitors of angiogenesis (development of new blood vessels).

Soybeans are a type of legume that can be eaten whole or processed into a variety of forms:

1. Whole Soy Products:

   Whole soy products are the least processed and include soybeans and edamame, which are immature (green) soybeans. Soy milk and tofu are also made from whole soybeans. Soy milk is made by soaking and grinding whole soybeans, boiling them in water and then filtering out the solids. It's commonly used as a milk alternative by people who cannot tolerate dairy or wish to avoid milk. Tofu is made by coagulating soy milk and pressing the curds into blocks. It's a common source of plant-based protein in vegetarian diets.

2. Fermented Soy:

   Fermented soy products are processed using traditional methods and include soy sauce, tempeh, miso and natto. Soy sauce is a liquid condiment made from fermented soy, roasted grains, salt water and a type of mold. Tempeh is a fermented soy cake that originated in Indonesia. Though not as popular as tofu, it's also commonly eaten as a source of protein in vegetarian diets.

3. Soy-Based Processed Foods:

   Soy is used to make several processed foods, including vegetarian and vegan meat substitutes, yogurts and cheeses. Soy flours, texturized vegetable protein and soybean oil are used in many packaged foods.

4. Soy Supplements:

   Soy protein isolate is a highly processed derivative of soy made by grinding soybeans into flakes and extracting the oil. The flakes are then mixed with alcohol or alkaline water, heated, and the resulting soy concentrate is spray-dried into a powder. Soy protein isolate is available in many protein powders and also added to many processed foods, such as protein bars and shakes. Other soy supplements include soy isoflavones, which are available in capsule form, and soy lecithin, which can be taken in capsules or as a powder.

Some medical experts argue soy has the following health benefits:

1. Eating soy is a great way to increase your plant protein. Research indicates that including more plant protein in your diet, as opposed to more carbohydrate, has clear cardiovascular benefits, such as lowering blood pressure.

2. Soy foods are naturally cholesterol-free and low in saturated fat. Animal protein foods high in saturated fat and cholesterol increase your risk of developing cardiovascular disease.

3. Substituting them with soy a few times each week can help cut saturated fats and reduce your overall risk for disease. See our table of savory soy protein substitutions.

4. Eating soy-based foods is a great way to boost your fiber intake. Fiber promotes a healthy gastrointestinal system, reduces cholesterol, and is associated with a reduced risk of developing cardiovascular disease. Including fiber-rich soy foods like edamame (green soybeans), black soybeans, soy nuts, soy flour and tempeh in your diet can help you boost your daily dietary fiber.

5. Soy foods are a good source of polyunsaturated fat. Polyunsaturated fats have a number of heart health benefits, such as lowering cholesterol. Choosing minimally processed soy foods will help you benefit from these heart-friendly fats.

6. Soy foods contain omega-3 fats, essential polyunsaturated fats. Omega-3 fats are linked to a lower risk of cardiovascular disease.

7. Soy foods are a great source of vitamins and minerals. B-vitamins, iron, zinc and an array of antioxidants round out the nutritional qualities of soy. In addition, many soy foods are enriched with vitamin B 12, calcium, and vitamin D to help vegetarians get these much-needed nutrients.

8.   Soy foods are a good source of phytochemicals. The phytochemicals in soy are called isoflavones. Isoflavones are currently being studied for their role in preventing postmenopausal bone loss and certain cancers.

9.   They believe soy contains prebiotic fiber and several beneficial phytochemicals, such as plant sterols

Contrary to popular belief, some experts point out that Asians consume approximately 2 teaspoons of soy on a daily basis. Experts believe oriental cultures consume mostly fermented soy products in smaller amounts such as: miso, tempeh, natto, shoyu, and tamari. Tofu is not fermented.

Some experts argue most modern soy food from soy milk are processed, which means they contain natural toxins called "antinutrients". These experts also argue that mega doses of phytoestrogens found in soy formulas are putting the normal sexual development of infants at risk. Soy-based infant formulas possibly contain the amount of estrogen in 5 birth control pills, which is believed to wreak havoc on the sexual development of babies.

Aside from containing antinutrients which are natural toxins, soy is believed to have a number of alarming compounds that may put your total health in peril.

1.   Soy contains goitrogens which lead to depressed thyroid function.

2.   It also contains phytates which prevent absorption of life enhancing minerals.

3.   It is also loaded with phytoestrogens which sometimes block the hormone estrogen and have adverse effects on human tissues.

A Summary of the Dangers of Soy:

1.   Soybeans and soy products contain high levels of phytic acid, which inhibits assimilation of calcium, magnesium, copper, iron, and zinc.

2.   Soaking, sprouting, and long, slow cooking do not neutralize phytic acid.

3.   Diets high in phytic acid have been shown to cause growth problems in children.

4.   Trypsin inhibitors in soy interfere with protein digestion and may cause pancreatic disorders.

5.   Test animals showed stunted growth when fed trypsin inhibitors from soy.

6.   The plant estrogens found in soy, called phytoestrogens, disrupt endocrine function, that is, the proper functioning of the glands that produce hormones, and have the potential to cause infertility as well as to promote breast cancer in adult women. Experts believe women trying to conceive should eat soy products in moderation because of their isoflavones. If over-consumed, isoflavones have different effects on a woman's body. Studies have shown that high levels of soy protein may increase menstrual cycle length and decrease FSH and luteinizing hormone levels. But no need to panic! Eating tofu will not make you infertile. Most people do not consume 60g of soy protein daily for over a month, which would generate this effect, according to research. Like with any food, eating in moderation and implementing a healthy food variety in your diet will ensure that you get all the important nutrients for your body without any adverse effects.

7.   Hypothyroidism and thyroid cancer may be caused by soy phytoestrogens.

8.   Infant soy formula has been linked to autoimmune thyroid disease.

9.   Soy has been found to increase the body's need for vitamin B12 and vitamin D.

10. Fragile soy proteins are exposed to high temperatures during processing in order to make soy protein isolate and textured vegetable protein, making them unsuitable for human digestion.

11. This same process results in the formation of toxic lysinoalanine and highly carcinogenic nitrosamines.

12. MSG, (also called free glutamic acid), a potent neurotoxin, is formed during soy food processing. Many soy products have extra MSG added as well.

13. Soy foods contain elevated levels of toxic aluminum, which negatively effects the nervous system the kidneys and has been implicated in the onset of Alzheimer's.

14. It's been found that babies given infant soy formulas have 13,000 to 22,000 times more estrogen than babies fed milk-based formulas.

15. Babies fed exclusively on infant soy formula are receiving the estrogenic equivalent (based on body weight) of at least four or five birth control pills per day! You read that right. Four or five birth control pills per day! By contrast, dairy-based infant formula contains almost no phytoestrogens, nor does human milk, even when the mother eats soy products.

16. There has been an increase of delayed physical maturation among boys, including lack of development of sexual organs.

17. Conversely, many girls today show signs of puberty, such as breast development and pubic hair, before the age of eight, and some even before the age of three.

18. Both of these abnormal conditions have been linked to the use of soy formulas as well as to exposure to "environmental estrogens" such as PCBs (polychlorinated biphenyls) and DDE (dichlorodiphenyl dichloroethylene) a breakdown product of DDT.

Some experts believe there are problems with soy protein isolate. Furthermore, modern soy foods are very different from those consumed traditionally in Asia. Most are made with soy protein isolate (SPI), which is a protein-rich powder extracted by an industrial process from the waste product of soy oil manufacturing. It is the industry's way of making a profit on a waste product. The industry spent over 30 years and billions of dollars developing SPI. In feeding studies, SPI caused many deficiencies in rats. That soy causes deficiencies in B12 and zinc is widely recognized, but the range of deficiencies was surprising. Although SPI is added to many foods, it was never granted GRAS status, meaning "Generally Recognized as Safe". The FDA only granted GRAS status to SPI for use as a binder in cardboard boxes. During the processing of soy, many additional toxins are formed, including nitrates (which are carcinogens) and a toxin called lysinoalanine. It was concerns about lysinoalanine in SPI that led the FDA to deny GRAS status for SPI as a food additive. In spite of all these dangers of soy protein isolate, SPI is the basic ingredient of soy infant formula. The FDA even allows a health claim for foods containing 6.25 grams SPI per serving.

Some experts believe the following medical conditions are possibly attributable to soy consumption:

1.   Asthma
2.   Chronic Fatigue
3.   Depression
4.   Diabetes
5.   Heart Arrhythmia
6.   Heart or Liver Disease
7.   Infertility/Reproductive Problems
8.   Irritable Bowel Syndrome
9.   Learning Disabilities/ADD/ADHD
10.   Pancreatic Disorders
11.   Premature or Delayed Puberty
12.   Rheumatoid Arthritis
13.   Thyroid Conditions: Auto-Immune Disorders (Graves' or Hashimoto's Disease), Goiter, Hypothyroidism, Thyroid Nodules, and Other thyroid disorders
14.   Uterine Cancer
15.   Weight Gain

Some experts believe if there is unhealthy soy, there is healthy soy. These experts believe fermented soy is healthy as opposed to unfermented soy. Some of these experts believe vitamin K2 is the forgotten vitamin found in these recommended fermented soy products. They believe vitamin K2 promotes heart health and gently redirects calcium back to your "bone bank". Some advocates of soy also believe that the nutritional benefits of soy depend on if it is processed or not. They believe the healthiest and most nutrient-rich form of soy is when it's unprocessed. They believe unprocessed soy contains all the essential amino acids—fiber, potassium, magnesium, B vitamins, calcium, iron—and the good fats, omega-3 and -6 fatty acids. In the United States, the majority of soy that is consumed is in the form of processed soy, which has less nutritional value. Some registered dietitians and health coaches recommend sticking with whole forms of soy, such as edamame, tofu, tempeh, and miso. She advises avoiding processed forms commonly used as "fillers" in snack foods and protein bars. They warn against other processed but popular foods, such as soy meats and cheeses. They also considers soy milk and soy flour healthy options and reinforces the approach of eating minimally processed, non-GMO sources of soy.

Some experts believe is a nutrient-dense food and an excellent alternative source of protein. The soybean contains all of the essential amino acids, as well as an impressive list of micronutrients (vitamins and minerals). Micronutrients in rich supply in soy include: calcium, iron, magnesium, manganese, phosphorus, potassium, vitamins B1, B2, B3, B5, B6, B9, C and zinc. Fiber and omega-3 and 6 fatty acids are also present in soy. These experts believe the composition of these nutrients varies among preparations but are in the highest quantity in whole soy foods such as edamame (whole soy beans), soy milk, tofu and tempeh.

Advocates of soy argue the following:

1. There is non-GMO soy available.
2. Misinformation regarding soy's relationship to cancer largely stems from confusion around the presence of phytoestrogens in soy. Phytoestrogen is not estrogen. Estrogen and testosterone are steroid hormones, and occur naturally in both sexes of humans, as well as in animals used for food. They help regulate sexual function and secondary sexual characteristics, in addition to nonsexual cellular functions. While estrogen plays many important beneficial roles in humans, it also naturally promotes proliferation of cells, and, at high levels, can

increase risk of some cancers by encouraging cells to multiply more than they usually would. Hormone replacement therapy in postmenopausal women (specifically, taking only estrogen) has also been implicated in cancer growth. While soy does not contain estrogen, animal foods do. Many consumers are aware that animals used for meat and dairy are commonly supplemented with synthetic growth hormones, but what they don't consider is that animal flesh and cow milk also contain their own naturally occurring estrogen— and this is true even of "grass-fed" and "organic" animals. Furthermore, meat, dairy and eggs all contain phytoestrogens; they are pervasive in our food, both plant and animal-derived, and you are not avoiding them entirely by avoiding soy. Phytoestrogen is just a catchall term for numerous naturally occurring plant compounds which are structurally similar to mammalian estrogen, and functionally are weakly estrogenic (weakly mimicking estrogen) or antiestrogenic (blocking estrogen's effects). The metabolism and functionality of phytoestrogens are incredibly complex and vary between individuals. The concern over soy and cancer stems from the fact that soy-based foods contain phytoestrogens (specifically, isoflavones) in varying amounts (depending on the preparation), and these react with the estrogen receptor. There are two types of estrogen receptors in humans: alpha and beta. Alpha are distributed widely throughout the body, whereas beta is localized in the ovary, prostate, lung, and epididymis (testicle). While isoflavones, like estrogen, bind to both alpha and beta receptors (preferentially to beta), isoflavones do not have the estrogenic effect of inducing tumor growth. In fact, isoflavones have demonstrated a protective benefit against hormone-dependent cancers. The inverse relationship between soy consumption and risk of developing premenopausal breast cancer has been clearly established. In other words, higher rates of soy intake are associated with lower rates of breast cancer. However, large clinical trials have not yet been conducted regarding the effect of phytoestrogen consumption on tumor growth in established cancer patients. To date, such studies have utilized small sample sizes, and the methods for obtaining data were highly variable. There have been 'promising' results from multiple animal models, demonstrating a reduction in tumor size with consumption of soy protein. Yet, aside from the immorality of artificially inducing cancer in unwilling participants, it is dangerous to compare laboratory animals to humans. We are not mice. Even within our species, there is tremendous variability in the metabolic processing of phytoestrogens and pharmacological agents, thus establishing the difficulty and complexity of this area of research. Instead, attention should be placed on the already available mass of epidemiological data which compares Asian cultures to those consuming a Western diet.

3. The relationship between soy consumption, iodine deficiency and goiter (enlarged thyroid) was first described in 1960 in The New England Journal of Medicine. Infants consuming nonfortified soy-based formula developed goiter, yet the exact nature of the relationship was unclear. Since then, there have been numerous studies which have disproven the causal relationship between soy and thyroid toxicity. TPO (thyroid peroxidase) is an enzyme located in the thyroid gland that catalyzes the necessary reactions to formulate thyroid hormone. Studies involving rats, pigs and humans demonstrated decreased TPO activity when fed isolated genistein and daidzein (the isoflavones in soy that react most strongly with TPO). Although some TPO activity was lost, there was no overall negative effect on thyroid function. Thyroid hormone levels measured in the blood of both experimental and control groups were the same. Furthermore, humans (as well as rats) only demonstrated hypothyroidism if their soy diets were iodine-depleted.

4. Whole soy foods are safe and nutritious. Advocates of soy recommend incorporating them into a diet which contains a good variety of fresh fruits and vegetables, grains and legumes.

5. Soy advocates believe soy is beneficial for your heart. They believe it can help lower blood pressure and cholesterol. They believe the fiber found in soy can help regulate blood sugar. They believe soy can aid in weight loss and prevent obesity.

Opponents of soy argue that soy contains chemicals that mimic estrogen and lower testosterone levels. These plant estrogens (phytoestrogens) cannot be wholly removed from any variety of soy food. The only way to remove the phytoestrogens is by alcohol extraction.

Soy contains protein. Soy is commonly referred to as meat without a bone. Soy is low in methionine, an essential sulphur-containing amino acid. Liver disease, brain disorders, osteoarthritis, fibromyalgia, chronic fatigue, and depression are just a few of the disorders that have responded to supplements of methionine. Soy, and many other foods, contain protease inhibitors, which interfere with the digestion of protein. Also, in order to prevent germination, phytates - which are found in beans, grains, and other seeds - tightly tie up minerals like calcium, zinc, and iron, which are essential for health and growth in children. Both protease inhibitors and phytates are greatly reduced by the traditional, time-consuming fermentation processes developed in the orient, but not by modern quick methods.

Lectins are proteins with a "sweet tooth." Found in beans, grains, and other foods they bite into carbohydrates, particularly sugars, often causing immune system reactions and blood clotting. Soybean lectins have two main functions. First, they react with the carbohydrate component of cell membranes, causing cell injuries and deaths. As this damage accumulates, it adversely affects the gastrointestinal, immune, and other systems of humans and other animal species. Second, they exist in a symbiotic relationship with Rhizobium bacteria. By fixing atmospheric nitrogen in the roots of the soybean plant, the lectin-bacteria team supports the miracle bean's traditional, historical use as a fertilizer and crop rotator.

Usually, soy lectins are digested and inactivated by traditional fermentation or by heat in soy processing. However, it has been found that "soybean meals can, on occasion, retain functional lectins at levels that may be detrimental to the animal's health and productivity. Soy protein intended for human consumption has consistently contained low levels of functionally intact lectins. This situation can be a problem for those people who eat large quantities of soy protein. Then, lectins are more than capable of perturbing digestive, absorptive, protective, and secretory functions throughout the gastrointestinal tract. Unlike ordinary food proteins, lectins strongly resist breakdown by enzymes in the gut. Again, lectins are not likely to be much of a problem if people only eat the soy protein infrequently and if they rotate their foods. However, some experts believe if you eat the soy protein regularly, as a principal source of protein, you are asking for problems from lectins and the many other anti-nutrients in soy.

Saponins are another anti-nutrient, along with protease inhibitors, phytates, and lectins, which all seem "to have evolved to help plants defend themselves against microbes, insects, and animal predators." Saponins injure the gut mucosa and contribute to "leaky gut syndrome." They are toxic to some fungi and yeasts and operate like the antifungal drug nystatin, which binds to the fungal cell membrane and increases its permeability. In the case of the drug, "side effects include pronounced damage to the patient's own cell membranes, with users complaining of gas, diarrhea, nausea, and stomach pain." People who consume modern soy foods complain of the same symptoms. Cooking and boiling do not remove saponins. "Only alcohol extraction removes them. When soy protein is removed from the oil, saponins stick with the protein." Fewer saponins are found in miso and tempeh. A bacterial enzyme, used in the fermentation that produces miso and tempeh, metabolizes and breaks down soy saponins. Saponins do lower cholesterol and may by themselves become a drug.

Soybeans contain goitrogens. Soy is not the only goitrogenic food. Broccoli, cabbage, Brussels sprouts, cassava, rapeseed, turnips, mustard, radish, peanuts, and millet also contain goitrogens. However, few adults-and even fewer children-eat these foods to excess. Furthermore, the goitrogens in most of these foods are easily neutralized by cooking or fermentation. Soy foods are different. The principal goitrogens in soybeans are the estrogenic plant hormones known as isoflavones. The antinutrients known as saponins in soy may also be goitrogens. Cooking and processing methods, using heat, pressure, and alkaline solutions, will neither deactivate nor remove isoflavones or saponins. Only solvent extraction can do that.

Cancer can be promoted by hormone mimickers, like the plant estrogens in soy.

In conclusion, I personally have this policy that if 2 or more reputable medical professionals corroborate a similar medical opinion, then I will follow their recommendations. If the edible item in question is not necessary to sustain human life, then I will abstain from eating this particular item.

This is why I eliminated soy and gluten from my personal diet. I would rather be safe than sorry.

I had to make a personal transition to give up fried foods. I can personally tell you it was one of the best decisions I have ever made. I don't regret it. I believe that if you decide to make this same decision and stick with it, you regret it either. I reduced my fried food intake. Then I stopped consuming fried foods altogether. This also includes "oven fried". I gradually weaned myself off of even organic "expeller pressed" foods.

Before the oil can be taken out of the oilseed, the seeds are first ground up into a paste. Next, those around up seeds a washed or purged with a solvent (also known as a petroleum distillate) such as hexane, to release the fat in the seed.

1. To remove that solvent from the oil, it is "flashed off" through heat in a sealed chamber. Then the oil/solvent blend is heated to approximately 212° F, distilling off the solvent and theoretically leaving virtually no detectable levels in the oil if the proper techniques have been applied. However, microscopic portions of up to 25 parts per million (25 ppm) of hexane can theoretically remain in the meal, which has been a point of high debate in the natural food industry.

2. Finally, that oil is then subject to the refining process, also known as "RBD" or Refined, Bleached & Deodorized in the industry. Some oil is also "degummed" and/or "winterized" as well. This is what makes canola oil have such a light color and flavor. It is also a similar process that occurs with soybean, sunflower, safflower, and refined olive oil.

3. Solvent expelling gets 97-99% of the oil out of the seed. It is the most efficient way to get all the oil from the canola seeds. That is one of the reasons that it is the cheapest canola option on the market.

Fried foods are unhealthy largely due to heated oils. Oil gets heated up to different temperatures during a cooking process. It is heated almost up to its smoking point for deep-frying and to lower temperatures for other types of cooking process. Oil starts to smoke when it is over-heated and starts to form aldehydes, ketones, alcohols, dienes, and acids. As a result, if you continue to cook something in the same oil, the food product will taste poorly. More importantly, the smoke of rapeseed, soybean, peanut oil and lard can cause serious mutagenicity and genetic toxicity. A few culprits to consider are an aldehyde called acrolein, as well as alkenals and alkadienals (unsaturated aldehydes) – they are formed during the burning/smoking process of the above-mentioned oil. There are quite a few fast food restaurants that use peanut oil to deep-fry their fries. Lard is widely used in pie crusts, and soybean is popular is households. Acrolien in very toxic to our cells and genes – they degrade our cells and genes; they also generate free radicals. Free radicals are responsible for cell aging. Recent studies have shown an increased amount of acrolein in Alzheimer's disease patients' brains. In a nutshell, oils with low smoking point (rapeseed, soybean, peanut oil, and lard) ⇒ acrolein ⇒ free radical ⇒ Alzheimer's disease + premature aging.

...

When you eat greasy food:

1. It strains your digestive system.
   When we eat greasy foods like fried food, the sheer   volume of fat puts a lot of pressure on our digestive system. Of fat, carbs and protein, fat is the most slowly digested, and it requires enzymes and digestive juices, like bile and stomach acid, to break it down. Everything from stress to medication can lower levels of these digestive juices, so many people are deficient to begin with. Add in fat, and your digestive system will be working overtime, often leading to bloating, nausea and discomfort.
2. It makes you run to the bathroom.

   The most common symptom of digestive strain is an unpleasant one. Not only will food just sit in your stomach, but it may enter the intestines inadequately digested. Sometimes you wind up seeing greasy or oily stools in these cases. Many people also experience diarrhea and stomach pain after eating greasy food.

3. It throws your gut bacteria out of whack.

More and more evidence suggest that what you eat affects your gut bacteria, also known as your microbiome. Greasy foods do not contain the nourishing, healthy fats that we find in things like avocados and fish. Eating more refined vegetable oils than nourishing fats tips the body's balance of fatty acids, which in turn may throw off everything from hormone levels to immune health.

4. Greasy food may cause acne.

   Greasy food likely does play a role in acne. The effect is indirect, occurring over time and as a result of a dietary pattern of eating. Acne is largely caused by hormonal imbalances and/or bacterial imbalances, so greasy foods cause acne by way of harming gut health.

5. It raises your risk for heart disease and diabetes.

   If your diet consistently includes greasy foods, you'll likely see your risk for chronic conditions—particularly heart disease—go up. A 2014 study from researchers at the Harvard T.H. Chan School of Public Health found that people who ate fried foods between four and six times per week saw their risk for Type 2 diabetes climb 39%, and their risk for coronary heart disease increase by 23%. For people who ate it every day, those percentages only got higher. Cardiovascular disease (CVD) is one of the leading major causes of morbidity and mortality worldwide. It may result from the interactions between multiple genetic and environmental factors including sedentary lifestyle and dietary habits. The quality of fats has been widely recognized to be inextricably linked to the pathogenesis of CVD. Vegetable oil is one of the essential dietary components in daily food consumption. However, the benefits of vegetable oil can be deteriorated by repeated heating that leads to lipid oxidation. The practice of using repeatedly heated cooking oil is not uncommon as it will reduce the cost of food preparation. Thermal oxidation yields new functional groups which may be potentially hazardous to cardiovascular health. Prolonged consumption of the repeatedly heated oil has been shown to increase blood pressure and total cholesterol, cause vascular inflammation as well as vascular changes which predispose to atherosclerosis. The harmful effect of heated oils is attributed to products generated from lipid oxidation during heating process. In view of the potential hazard of oxidation products, therefore this review article will provide an insight and awareness to the general public on the consumption of repeatedly heated oils which is detrimental to health.

6. Fried foods increase your risk of developing Alzheimer's disease.

In terms of brain danger, eating too much fried food is related to saturated fat and cholesterol. The saturated fat in fried food is shown to damage the blood-brain barrier. One interesting observation from animal models is that it seems that diets higher in saturated fats disrupt the blood-barrier. The barrier is a complex transport system for nutrients into the brain. When it's disrupted, it can allow harmful substances to get in and perhaps injure the brain. It can also disrupt the uptake of nutrients that are important for brain function. In addition, fried food is also known to increase blood cholesterol levels. Cholesterol is a central dietary component in the development of Alzheimer's disease. There's a link between blood cholesterol levels and dementia. A 2014 study in the Journal of the American Medical Association revealed that people who have high levels of bad (LDL) cholesterol and low levels of good cholesterol (HDL) are more likely to have a build-up of beta-amyloid proteins in their brain, which are harbingers of Alzheimer's disease and dementia. More research needs to be conducted to figure out whether high cholesterol is a cause or a result of Alzheimer's progression.

7. Trans-fats hurt brain function and memory.
While the FDA aims to completely eradicate trans-fats from the food supply, many foods still contain a hefty amount of this damaging fat, which remains solid at room temperature. The top offenders right now include stick margarine, frosting, frozen pizza, refrigerated dough, coffee creamer, and microwave popcorn. A 2011 study in the journal Neurology exposed two scary consequences of eating too much trans-fat: less favorable cognitive function and less total cerebral brain volume. Though experts believe more studies are needed to confirm the role trans-fat plays in brain health, the well-established dangers of trans-fats

should be enough motivation to kick the stuff. In an analysis of 50 studies on trans-fats, a recent review found that high-trans-fat diets raise your risk of dying from heart disease by 28 percent, and from any cause by 34 percent. Eating a high trans-fat diet will increase bad cholesterol and decrease good cholesterol. In one study, we found that even a moderate intake of trans-fat is worse than a high intake of saturated fats.

Expeller pressed oil means that the oil was mechanically extracted with a screw press. This traditional way of making oil is much healthier than using hexane – but the big oil manufacturers don't like this method because it's less effective (less oil is made) and it's more expensive. So, it's used less often. The expeller pressing process can cause a lot of heat that can make the oil go rancid, so some companies take it step farther and cold press their oils at temps of no more than 80°F to 120°F, which is labor intensive but produces the best oils. Beware that although the term "cold pressed" is regulated in Europe, it's not very well regulated in the U.S. and cold pressed oils could technically be made at high temperatures – so I don't take this term on a label at face value.

As I informed you earlier, I eventually weaned myself off of even expeller pressed foods. I was told that expeller pressed foods are technically still considered fried foods, but just fried at a lower temperature. Some experts believe foods cooked in expeller pressed oil is healthier than foods cooked in conventional oil.

How expeller pressed oil is made:

1. Expelled pressing uses a press to physically squeeze the oil out of the seed, rather than use chemicals. With this method, no solvents are used in the process, and therefore don't have the chance of having any hexane residue left over.

2. An expeller press is a screw type machine which presses oil through a caged barrel-like-cavity, using friction and continuous pressure. The screw drives forward to literally squeeze the oil from the compressed

seeds. There isn't any added heat in this process, but the pressure and friction involved in the pressing process creased heat from the unit in the range of 140-210° F. So technically, this process is not "cold pressed".

3. After the oil is removed, the remaining seed solids are left over forming a hardened cake, which is removed and later sold as meal for animal feed. Expeller pressing gets 87-95% of the oil out of the seed, so there is some oil still left over after pressing (though some claim as little as 65% is removed, so this is debated). Therefore, this option is not the cheapest, which can make this oil more expensive than the solvent expelled standard.

4. Expeller pressed oil is typically refined (or RBD) using the same process as described above. This refining process involves additional heat from steam and the use of a natural earthen bleaching clay.

How cold pressed oil is made:

1. Cold pressed seed oils must be produced below 122° F (as is legally defined in Europe) and should only apply to fully unrefined oils that are not heated later during the refining process.

2. The term "cold pressed" has sometimes been improperly used to describe expeller pressed oils, but these are really two different things. Cold pressing typically involves one of the following methods.

3. The ancient method of stone grinding or milling, as in the crushing of olive oils (quite an outdated method for any bulk EVOO production)

4. Bladder press extraction, which use simple compression for fruit oils such as olive and avocado. Hydraulic presses, which use simple slow compression.

5. Low resistance expeller pressing, which is done at a very slow rate to not exceed 122° F.

6.   Modified Atmospheric Crushing (MAC) and Modified Atmospheric Packing (MAP), which employ enhanced cooling and refrigeration techniques using modified vegetable oil expeller presses that meet cold pressing temperature standards.

7.   Remember that when related to most Extra Virgin Olive Oil, that is actually "cold spun" using a centrifuge in today's market.

8.   The cold pressing process typically removes the least amount from the oil from the seed, making it the least efficient and the most expensive process available.

Chapter 10

No Fried Food

Towards the end of chapter 10, we discussed the dangers of heated oils with regard to fried foods. Fried foods are high in unhealthy fat and calories. A few studies, including one published in 2014, have linked fried foods to serious health problems like type 2 diabetes and heart disease. Fried foods may influence risk of these diseases through several key risk factors: obesity, high blood pressure, and high cholesterol. The process of frying is known to alter the quality and increase the caloric content of food. Prior to the current trans-fat ban, fried foods served in fast-food restaurants were often cooked in hydrogenated oils high in trans fats. Trans fats raise bad (LDL) cholesterol levels, lower good (HDL) cholesterol levels, and raise your chance of having heart disease.

Fried foods for the most part are defined as foods cooked in oil or any other fluid(s) apart from water. From shallow frying to deep frying, there are so many different ways to fry:

1. **Shallow Frying:**
    Shallow frying is frying over a high heat using a small amount of oil.

2. **Deep Frying:**
    Deep frying entails frying food fully immersed in oil.

3. **Stir-Frying:**
    Stir fry is frying different ingredients in very hot oil, while stirring constantly. Only a small amount of oil is required for a stir-fry.

4. **Sautéing:**
    Sautéing requires keeping the ingredients moving around in the pan, either by using a wooden spoon or by moving the pan back and forth.

Most cooking oils go through an insane amount of processing with chemical solvents, steamers, neutralizers, de-waxers, bleach and deodorizers before they end up in the bottle. The "solvent" that is most often used to extract the oil is the neurotoxin hexane – and it's literally bathed in it. Hexane is a cheap byproduct from gasoline production, that's a serious occupational hazard and toxic air pollutant. It's been shown that some hexane residue can remain in the oil, and the FDA doesn't require food manufacturers to test for residues. Residue tests done as a part of research in 2009 found hexane residues in soybean oil. So, you very well could be eating this chemical every time we cook with hexane-extracted oils. Almost all toxicology research focuses on the industrial use and inhalation of hexane, so no one knows exactly how dangerous eating it is – but it surely isn't healthy. Two well renown cooking oils companies openly admitted to using GMOs and hexane extraction in their processing.

Oil facts:

1. Canola Oil – To better understand this oil, it helps to know where it comes from. Canola oil is extracted from rapeseed plants, that have been bred to have lower levels of toxic erucic acid. Before it was bred this way, it was called Rapeseed Oil and used for industrial purposes because the erucic acid in it caused heart damage in animal studies. It got the fancy new name "canola", but it still contains trace amounts of erucic acid (up to 2%, which they consider "safe"). In 1995 they also began genetically engineering (GMO) rapeseed to be resistant to herbicides, and now almost all canola crops in North America are GMO. Canola oil consumption has been linked to vitamin E deficiency and a shortened life span in animal studies. Research has also found some trans fats in canola oil, which were created during the heavy processing that it goes through. These trans fats are not labeled. This is ironic because trans fats are the opposite of heart healthy! Like all modern vegetable oils, canola oils undergo the process of caustic refining, bleaching, and degumming. All of this processing involves high temperatures or chemicals of questionable safety. Canola oil contains omega 3 fatty acids. Omega 3 fatty acids can become rancid when exposed to oxygen at high temperatures; it must be deodorized.

The standard deodorization process removes a large portion of the omega 3 fatty acids by turning them into trans fatty acids. These trans fatty acids are not on the label.

2. Cottonseed Oil – It's a byproduct of the cotton crop that's inundated with pesticides and chemicals because it's regulated as a textile crop – not food! Cotton farming also may be killing India's farmers, as harsh pesticides sicken them and thousands more have committed suicide – many after the costly GMO seeds they used failed. Cottonseed oil does not belong in our food supply and should be strictly avoided. Thankfully, most cooking oils in the grocery store no longer contain cottonseed oil, and this ingredient is mostly relegated to the processed food aisle. Cottonseed is widely being replaced in cooking oils with another oil that I avoid: soybean oil.

3. Soybean Oil – Most products that just say "Vegetable Oil" are made from soybeans. It's so common in processed foods that up to 20% of calories in the typical American diet is thought to come from soybean oil. Soybean oil is high in omega-6 fatty acids, and our bodies need this type of fatty acid, but today people are getting too much of it through processed foods – up to 20 times more than required, according to some estimates. The overabundance of omega-6 fatty acids increases the risk of inflammation, cardiovascular disease, cancer, and autoimmune diseases. Soybean oil is also typically made from GMOs, as 94% of U.S. soybean crops are genetically modified. A recent survey showed that the most widely utilized vegetable oil in America, is now made from soybeans (previously cottonseed). This company donated over $2.6 million dollars to fight GMO labeling laws in the U.S. Every time you buy their products you help fund these anti-labeling campaigns. Other cooking oils that are often extracted with hexane and are high in omega-6 fatty acids include sunflower and safflower.

4. Corn Oil – A larger cooking oil company recently claimed that corn oil lowers cholesterol better than olive oil? This company partially funded the study that supported this claim. The truth that they don't mention in their commercials is that corn oil is highly refined, hexane-extracted from GMO corn, and loaded with omega-6 polyunsaturated fatty acids that are unstable when exposed to heat. This instability causes oxidation, a

process that generates free radicals. Free radicals are renegade molecules in the body that damage cells, triggering a host of diseases from liver damage to cancer. This company also confirmed that their cooking oils are made from GMOs (corn, soybean, canola) and that they use hexane extraction for all oils, except for their olive oils.

Cooking oils have smoke points. The smoke point of an oil is exactly what it sounds like: the point at which an oil begins to smoke. The smoke point is a natural property of unrefined oils, reflecting an oil's chemical composition. One of the main reasons for refining (or processing) an oil is to raise its smoke point. When an oil is heated past its smoke point, it generates toxic fumes and free radicals which are extremely harmful to your body. When the smoke point is reached, you'll begin to see the gaseous vapors from heating, a marker that the oil has started to decompose. Decomposition involves chemical changes that not only negatively affect the food's flavor and nutritional value, but also create cancer-causing compounds that are harmful when consumed and/or inhaled. You want to keep these vapors out of your lungs. You want to definitely throw away the food that has been in contact with this oil to deter or prevent free radicals from entering your body.

Below is a table that lists various cooking oils, their smoke points, and Omega-6 and Omega-3 ratios.

Cooking Oils / Fats	Smoke Point °C	Smoke Point °F	Omega-6: Omega-3 Ratio (plus other relevant fat information)
Unrefined flaxseed oil	107°C	225°F	1:4
Unrefined safflower oil	107°C	225°F	133:1
Unrefined sunflower oil	107°C	225°F	40:1
Unrefined corn oil	160°C	320°F	83:1
Unrefined high-oleic sunflower oil	160°C	320°F	40:1, 84% monosaturated
Extra virgin olive oil	160°C	320°F	73% monounsaturated, high in Omega 9
Unrefined peanut oil	160°C	320°F	32:1

Semi refined safflower oil	160°C	320°F	133:1, (75% Omega 9)
Unrefined soy oil	160°C	320°F	8:1 (most are GMO)
Unrefined walnut oil	160°C	320°F	5:1
Hemp seed oil	165°C	330°F	3:1
Butter	177°C	350°F	9:1, Mostly saturated & monosaturated
Semi refined canola oil	177°C	350°F	2:1 [(56% Omega 9), 80% Canola is GMO.]
Coconut oil	177°C	350°F	86% healthy saturated, lauric acid (has antibacterial, antioxidant, and antiviral properties). Contains 66% medium chain triglycerides (MCTs).
Unrefined sesame oil	177°C	350°F	138:1

Semi refined soy oil	177°C	350°F	8:1
Vegetable shortening	182°C	360°F	mostly unhealthy saturated, Trans Fat
Lard	182°C	370°F	11:1 high in saturated
Macadamia nut oil	199°C	390°F	1:1, 80% monounsaturated, (83% Omega-9)
Canola oil (Expeller Pressed)	200°C	400°F	2:1, 62% monounsaturated, 32% polyunsaturated
Refined canola oil	204°C	400°F	3:1, 80% of Canola in US in GMO.
Semi refined walnut oil	204°C	400°F	5:1
High quality (low acidity) extra virgin olive oil	207°C	405°F	13:1, 74% monosaturated (71.3% Omega 9)

Sesame oil	210°C	410°F	42:1
Cottonseed oil	216°C	420°F	54:1
Grapeseed oil	216°C	420°F	676:1, (12% saturated, 17% monounsaturated)
Virgin olive oil	216°C	420°F	13:1, 74% monosaturated (71.3% Omega 9)
Almond oil	216°C	420°F	Omega-6 only
Hazelnut oil	221°C	430°F	75% monosaturated (no Omega 3, 78% Omega 9)
Peanut oil	227°C	440°F	32:1
Sunflower oil	227°C	440°F	40:1
Refined corn oil	232°C	450°F	83:1
Palm oil	232°C	450°F	46:1, mostly saturated and monosaturated

Palm kernel oil	232°C	450°F	82% saturated (No Omega 3)
Refined high-oleic sunflower oil	232°C	450°F	39:1, 84% monosaturated
Refined peanut oil	232°C	450°F	32:1
Semi refined sesame oil	232°C	450°F	138:1
Refined soy oil	232°C	450°F	8:1 (most are GMO)
Semi refined sunflower oil	232°C	450°F	40:1
Olive pomace oil	238°C	460°F	74% monosaturated, high in Omega 9
Extra light olive oil			
Ghee			

(Clarified Butter)	242°C	468°F	74% monosaturated, high in Omega 9
	252°C	485°F	0:0, 62% saturated fat
Rice Bran Oil	254°C	490°F	21:1, Good source of vitamin E & antioxidants
Refined Safflower oil	266°C	510°F	133:1 (74% Omega 9)
Avocado oil	271°C	520°F	12:1, 70% monosaturated, (68% Omega-9 fatty acids) High in vitamin E.

Another worry with fried food centers on acrylamide, a chemical that forms in foods cooked at high temperatures, such as fried and baked foods. Acrylamide has been shown in animal studies to cause cancer. When food is cooked at very high heat, an amino acid -- asparagine -- in the food reacts with sugars to produce acrylamide. This chemical can form in many fried foods, but it's especially common in potatoes, which are high in sugars like fructose and glucose. The darker the food, the more acrylamide there is. If you have a family history of cancer, you need to be conscious of how many fried foods you eat.

Acrylamide is a chemical used mainly in certain industrial processes, such as in making paper, dyes, and plastics, and in treating drinking water and wastewater. There are small amounts in some consumer products, such as caulk, food packaging, and some adhesives. Acrylamide is also found in cigarette smoke. Acrylamide can also form in some starchy foods during high-temperature cooking, such as frying, roasting, and baking. Acrylamide forms from sugars and an amino acid that are naturally in food; it does not come from food packaging or the environment.

Acrylamide doesn't appear to be in raw foods themselves. It's formed when certain starchy foods are cooked at high temperatures (above about 250° F). Cooking at high temperatures causes a chemical reaction between certain sugars and an amino acid (asparagine) in the food, which forms acrylamide. Cooking methods such as frying, baking, broiling, or roasting are more likely to create acrylamide, while boiling and steaming appear less likely to do so. Longer cooking times and cooking at higher temperatures can increase the amount of acrylamide in foods further. Acrylamide is found mainly in plant foods, such as potato products, grain products, or coffee. Foods such as French fries and potato chips seem to have the highest levels of acrylamide, but it's also found in breads and other grain products. Acrylamide does not form (or forms at lower levels) in dairy, meat, and fish products.

Acrylamide is also found in cigarette smoke. This is probably one of the major ways smokers are exposed. People who work in certain industries (particularly in the paper and pulp, construction, foundry, oil drilling, textiles, cosmetics, food processing, plastics, mining, and agricultural industries) may be exposed to acrylamide in the workplace, mainly through skin contact or by breathing it in. Regulations limit exposure in these settings.

Researchers use 2 main types of studies to try to figure out if a substance causes cancer:

1. Lab studies: In these studies, animals are exposed to a substance (often in very large doses) to see if it causes tumors or other health problems. Researchers might also expose normal cells in a lab dish to the substance to see if it causes the types of changes that are seen in cancer cells. It's not always clear if the results from these types of studies will apply to humans, but lab studies are a good way to find out if a substance might possibly cause cancer.

2. Studies in people: This type of study looks at cancer rates in different groups of people. It might compare the cancer rate in a group exposed to a substance to the cancer rate in a group not exposed to it or compare it to the cancer rate in the general population. But sometimes it can be hard to know what the results of these studies mean, because many other factors might affect the results.

In most cases neither type of study provides enough evidence on its own, so researchers usually look at both lab-based and human studies when trying to figure out if something causes cancer. Based on the studies done so far, it's not yet clear if acrylamide affects cancer risk in people.

Acrylamide has been found to increase the risk of several types of cancer when given to lab animals (rats and mice) in their drinking water. The doses of acrylamide given in these studies have been as much as 1,000 to 10,000 times higher than the levels people might be exposed to in foods. It's not clear if these results would apply to people as well, but in general it makes sense to limit human exposure to substances that cause cancer in animals.

Since acrylamide was first found in certain foods in 2002, dozens of studies have looked at whether people who eat more of these foods might be at higher risk for certain cancers. Most of the studies done so far have not found an increased risk of cancer in humans. For some types of cancer, such as kidney, endometrial, and ovarian cancer, the results have been mixed, but there are currently no cancer types for which there is clearly an increased risk related to acrylamide intake.

The studies that have been done so far have had some important limits. For example, many of the studies relied on food questionnaires that people filled out every couple of years. These questionnaires might not have accounted for all dietary sources of acrylamide. In addition, people might not accurately remember what they have eaten when asked in personal interviews or through questionnaires. While the evidence from human studies so far is somewhat reassuring, more studies are needed to determine if acrylamide raises cancer risk in people. The American Cancer Society supports the call by federal and international agencies for continued evaluation of how acrylamide is formed, its health risks, and how its presence in food can be reduced or removed.

Several national and international agencies study substances in the environment to determine if they can cause cancer. (A substance that causes cancer or helps cancer grow is called a *carcinogen*.) The American Cancer Society looks to these organizations to evaluate the risks based on evidence from laboratory, animal, and human research studies. The International Agency for Research on Cancer (IARC) is part of the World Health Organization (WHO). Its major goal is to identify causes of cancer. IARC classifies acrylamide as a "probable human carcinogen" based on data showing it can increase the risk of some types of cancer in lab animals. The evidence in humans was considered to be "inadequate" at the time of the last IARC review of the subject (1994), and at that time acrylamide was not known to be found in foods.

The National Toxicology Program (NTP) is formed from parts of several different US government agencies, including the National Institutes of Health (NIH), the Centers for Disease Control and Prevention (CDC), and the Food and Drug Administration (FDA). In its most recent *Report on Carcinogens* (2014), the NTP has classified acrylamide as "reasonably anticipated to be a human carcinogen" based on the studies in lab animals. The US Environmental Protection Agency (EPA) maintains the Integrated Risk Information System (IRIS), an electronic database that contains information on human health effects from exposure to various substances in the environment. The EPA classifies acrylamide as "likely to be carcinogenic to humans" based on studies in lab animals.

It's important to note that the determinations above are based mainly on studies in lab animals, and not on studies of people's exposure to acrylamide from foods. Since the discovery of acrylamide in foods, the American Cancer Society, the FDA, and many other organizations have recognized the need for further research on this topic. Ongoing studies will continue to provide new information on whether acrylamide levels in foods are linked to increased cancer risk.

In the United States, the FDA regulates the amount of residual acrylamide in a variety of materials that come in contact with food, but there are currently no regulations on the presence of acrylamide in food itself. In 2016, the FDA issued guidance to help the food industry reduce the amount of acrylamide in certain foods, but these are recommendations, not regulations. The EPA regulates acrylamide in drinking water. The EPA has set an acceptable level of acrylamide exposure, which is low enough to account for any uncertainty in the data relating acrylamide to cancer and other health effects. In the workplace, exposure to acrylamide is regulated by the EPA and the Occupational Safety and Health Administration (OSHA).

For most people, the major potential sources of acrylamide exposure are in certain foods and in cigarette smoke. It's not yet clear if the levels of acrylamide in foods raise cancer risk, but for people who are concerned, there are some things you can do to lower your exposure.

Certain foods are more likely to contain acrylamide than others. These include potato products (especially French fries and potato chips), coffee, and foods made from grains (such as breakfast cereals, cookies, and toast). These foods are often part of a regular diet. But if you want to lower your acrylamide intake, reducing your intake of these foods is one way to do so.

The FDA's advice on acrylamide is to adopt a healthy eating plan, consistent with the Dietary Guidelines for Americans, that:

1. Emphasizes fruits, vegetables, whole grains, and fat-free or low-fat milk and milk products.

2. Includes lean meats, poultry, fish, beans, eggs, and nuts.

3. Is low in saturated fats, trans fats, cholesterol, salt (sodium), and added sugars.

This type of diet is likely to have health benefits beyond lowering acrylamide levels.

Acrylamide has been detected in both home-cooked and in packaged or processed foods. Acrylamide levels in foods can vary widely depending on the manufacturer, the cooking time, and the method and temperature of the cooking process. Since acrylamide is formed from natural chemicals in food during cooking, acrylamide levels in cooked organic foods are likely to be similar to levels in cooked non-organic foods.

For potatoes, frying causes the highest acrylamide formation. Roasting potato pieces causes less acrylamide formation, followed by baking whole potatoes. Boiling potatoes with skin on does not create acrylamide. Soaking raw potato slices in water for 15 to 30 minutes before frying or roasting helps reduce acrylamide formation during cooking. (Soaked potatoes should be drained and blotted dry before cooking to prevent splattering or fires.) Storing potatoes in the refrigerator can result in increased acrylamide during cooking. Therefore, store potatoes outside the refrigerator, preferably in a dark, cool place, such as a closet or a pantry, to prevent sprouting. Generally, acrylamide levels rise when cooking is done for longer periods or at higher temperatures. Cooking cut potato products, such as frozen French fries or potato slices, to a golden yellow color rather than a brown color helps reduce acrylamide formation. Brown areas tend to have more acrylamide.

Toasting bread to a light brown color, rather than a dark brown color, lowers the amount of acrylamide. Very brown areas contain the most acrylamide. Acrylamide forms in coffee when coffee beans are roasted, not when coffee is brewed at home or in a restaurant. So far, scientists have not found good ways to reduce acrylamide formation in coffee. Not smoking and avoiding secondhand smoke are other ways to potentially reduce your exposure to acrylamide, as well as to many other potentially harmful chemicals.

Some experts believe that enzymes commonly found within the vegetables and possibly fruits can break down acrylamide or prevent it from wreaking havoc internally.

Chapter 11

6:00 a.m. — 6:00 p.m.

UPDATE

At the beginning of Chapter 7: Organic and Natural Supplements, I informed readers of my recent practice of taking my vitamins and or supplements at night time before sleep for better or increased absorption. Despite this recent practice, I still practice intermittent fasting. I am an early bird, who likes to get up early in the morning. I also believe in the nutritional importance of consuming breakfast.

Mondays thru Fridays, I eat a larger meal during earlier morning hours then I typically practice intermittent fasting throughout the day until it is time for me to take my vitamins and or supplements at night time (with the exception of drinking water throughout the day for hydration purposes).

On the weekends, I will still eat a larger meal during morning hours and possibly snack on 1 smaller portion of either cashews, pecans, or almonds after exercising until I take vitamins and or supplements at night time. On the weekends, I also drink water throughout the day for hydration purposes.

I still practice no food and or beverage intake from 6:00 p.m. until 6:00 a.m. (with the exception of the vitamins and or supplements I consume at night before sleep with aloe vera juice).

I remember when I first made the decision not to eat any food or to drink any beverage except water from 6:00 p.m. to 6:00 a.m. I remember not being able to wait until 6:00 a.m. However, this went away as I decided to stick with it.

Intermittent fasting is the ancient secret of health. It is ancient because it has been practiced throughout all of human history. It's a secret because this powerful habit has been virtually forgotten. But now many people are re-discovering this dietary intervention. It can carry huge benefits if it is done right: weight loss, increased energy, reversal of type 2 diabetes and many other things. Plus, you'll *save* time and money.

Intermittent fasting is not starvation, but more so self-restraint or self-constraint. Starvation is defined as the involuntary absence of food. Starvation is neither deliberate or controlled in most cases. Fasting is the voluntary withholding of food. Fasting simply allows the body to burn off excess body fat. It is important to realize that this is normal and humans have evolved to fast without detrimental health consequences. Body fat is merely food energy that has been stored away. If you don't eat, your body will simply "eat" its own fat for energy. When we eat, more food energy is ingested than can immediately be used. Some of this energy must be stored away for later use. Insulin is the key hormone involved in the storage of food energy.

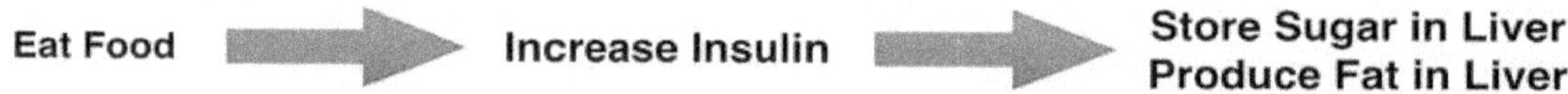

Insulin rises when we eat, helping to store the excess energy in two separate ways. Sugars can be linked into long chains, called glycogen and then stored in the liver. There is, however, limited storage space; and once that is reached, the liver starts to turn the excess glucose into fat. This process is called De-Novo Lipogenesis (meaning literally Making Fat from New). Some of this newly created fat is stored in the liver, but most of it is exported to other fat deposits in the body. While this is a more complicated process, there is no limit to the amount of fat that can be created. So, two complementary food energy storage systems exist in our bodies. One is easily accessible but with limited storage space (glycogen), and the other is more difficult to access but has unlimited storage space (body fat).

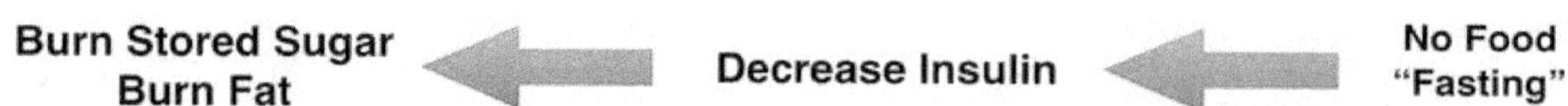

The process goes in reverse when we do not eat (intermittent fasting). Insulin levels fall, signaling the body to start burning stored energy as no more is coming through food. Blood glucose falls, so the body must now pull glucose out of storage to burn for energy. Glycogen is the most easily accessible energy source. It is broken down into glucose molecules to provide energy for the other cells. This can provide enough energy to power the body for 24-36 hours. After that, the body will start breaking down fat for energy. So, that the body only really exists in two states – the fed (insulin high) state and the fasted (insulin low) state. Either we are storing food energy, or we are burning it. It's one or the other. If eating and fasting are balanced, then there is no net weight gain.

If we start eating the minute we roll out of bed, and do not stop until we go to sleep, we spend almost all our time in the fed state. Over time, we will gain weight. We have not allowed our body any time to burn food energy. To restore balance or to lose weight, we simply need to increase the amount of time we burn food energy. That's intermittent fasting. In essence, fasting allows the body to use its stored energy.

Some benefits of intermittent fasting:

1. Improved mental clarity and concentration
2. Weight and body fat loss
    (Fasting increases basal metabolic rate.)
3. Lowered blood insulin and sugar levels
4. Possible reversal of type 2 diabetes
5. Increased energy
6. Improved fat burning
7. Increased growth hormone
8. Lowering blood cholesterol
9. Possible prevention of Alzheimer's disease
10. Longer longevity
11. Activation of cellular cleansing
12. Inflammation reduction

Intermittent fasting changes the function of cells, genes and hormones. A lot of the benefits of intermittent fasting are related to these changes in hormones, gene expression and function of cells. When you don't eat for a while, several things happen in your body. For example, your body initiates important cellular repair processes and changes hormone levels to make stored body fat more accessible.

Here are some of the changes that occur in your body during fasting:

1.   Insulin levels: Blood levels of insulin drop significantly, which facilitates fat burning.

2.   Human growth hormone: The blood levels of growth hormone may increase as much as 5-fold. Higher levels of this hormone facilitate fat burning and muscle gain and have numerous other benefits.

3.   Cellular repair: The body induces important cellular repair processes, such as removing waste material from cells.

4.   Gene expression: There are beneficial changes in several genes and molecules related to longevity and protection against disease.

Intermittent fasting induces various cellular repair processes. When we fast, the cells in the body initiate a cellular "waste removal" process called autophagy. This involves the cells breaking down and metabolizing broken and dysfunctional proteins that build up inside cells over time. Increased autophagy may provide protection against several diseases, including cancer and Alzheimer's disease.

Intermittent fasting can help you lose weight and belly fat. Generally speaking, intermittent fasting will make you eat fewer meals. Unless if you compensate by eating much more during the other meals, you will end up taking in fewer calories. Additionally, intermittent fasting enhances hormone function to facilitate weight loss. Lower insulin levels, higher growth hormone levels and increased amounts of norepinephrine (noradrenaline) all increase the breakdown of body fat and facilitate its use for energy. For this reason, short-term fasting actually increases your metabolic rate by 3.6-14%, helping you burn even more calories. In other words, intermittent fasting works on both sides of the calorie equation. It boosts your metabolic rate (increases calories out) and reduces the amount of food you eat (reduces calories in).

Intermittent fasting can reduce insulin resistance, lowering Your risk of type 2 diabetes. Type 2 diabetes main feature is high blood sugar levels in the context of insulin resistance. Anything that reduces insulin resistance should help lower blood sugar levels and protect against type 2 diabetes. Interestingly, intermittent fasting has been shown to have major benefits for insulin resistance and lead to an impressive reduction in blood sugar levels. One study in diabetic rats also showed that intermittent fasting protected against kidney damage, one of the most severe complications of diabetes. However, there may be some differences between genders. One study in women showed that blood sugar control actually worsened after a 22-day long intermittent fasting protocol. This is probably why some experts recommend intermittent fasts for women not to exceed 14 to 15 hours at a time.

ntermittent fasting can reduce oxidative stress and inflammation in the body. Oxidative stress is one of the steps towards aging and many chronic diseases. It involves unstable molecules called free radicals, which react with other important molecules (like protein and DNA) and damage them. Several studies show that intermittent fasting may enhance the body's resistance to oxidative stress. Additionally, studies show that intermittent fasting can help fight inflammation, another key driver of all sorts of common diseases.

Intermittent fasting may be beneficial for heart health. It is known that various health markers (so-called "risk factors") are associated with either an increased or decreased risk of heart disease. Intermittent fasting has been shown to improve numerous different risk factors, including blood pressure, total and LDL cholesterol, blood triglycerides, inflammatory markers and blood sugar levels. However, a lot of this is based on animal studies. The effects on heart health need to be studied a lot further in humans before recommendations can be made.

Intermittent fasting may help prevent cancer. Cancer is characterized by uncontrolled growth of cells. Fasting has been shown to have several beneficial effects on metabolism that may lead to reduced risk of cancer. Although human studies are needed, promising evidence from animal studies indicates that intermittent fasting may help prevent cancer. There is also some evidence on human cancer patients, showing that fasting reduced various side effects of chemotherapy.

Intermittent fasting is good for your brain. What is good for the body is often good for the brain as well. Intermittent fasting improves various metabolic features known to be important for brain health. This includes reduced oxidative stress, reduced inflammation and a reduction in blood sugar levels and insulin resistance. Several studies in rats have shown that intermittent fasting may increase the growth of new nerve cells, which should have benefits for brain function. It also increases levels of a brain hormone called brain-derived neurotrophic factor (BDNF), a deficiency of which has been implicated in depression and various other brain problems. Animal studies have also shown that intermittent fasting protects against brain damage due to strokes.

Intermittent fasting may help prevent Alzheimer's disease. Alzheimer's disease is the world's most common neurodegenerative disease. A study in rats shows that intermittent fasting may delay the onset of Alzheimer's disease or reduce its severity. In a series of case reports, a lifestyle intervention that included daily short-term fasts was able to significantly improve Alzheimer's symptoms in 9 out of 10 patients. Animal studies also suggest that fasting may protect against other neurodegenerative diseases, including Parkinson's and Huntington's disease. However, more research in humans is needed.

Intermittent fasting may extend your lifespan, helping you live longer. One of the most exciting applications of intermittent fasting may be its ability to extend lifespan. Studies in rats have shown that intermittent fasting extends lifespan in a similar way as continuous calorie restriction. In some of these studies, the effects were quite dramatic. In one of them, rats that fasted every other day lived 83% longer than rats who weren't fasted.

Fasting offers infinite flexibility. You can fast for as long or short as you like, but here are some popular regimens. Generally, shorter fasts are done more frequently.

Types of intermittent fasts:

- Keto and intermittent fasting: "I am completely blown away by the changes"

- Intermittent fasting: down 42 pounds in 14 months

- How Gino reversed his type 2 diabetes by doing the opposite

1. Shorter fasts (<24hrs)
   a. 16:8: This way of doing intermittent fasting involves daily fasting for 16 hours. Sometimes this is also referred to as an 8-hour eating 'window'. You eat all your meals within an 8-hour time period and fast for the remaining 16 hours. Generally, this is done daily or almost daily. For example, you may eat all your meals within the time period of 11:00 am and 7:00 pm. Generally, this means skipping breakfast. You generally eat two or three meals within this 8-hour period. This method is also known as the Leangains protocol. Doing this method of fasting can actually be as simple as not eating anything after dinner and skipping breakfast. It is generally recommended that women only fast 14-15 hours, because they seem to do better with slightly shorter fasts. For people who get hungry in the morning and like to eat breakfast, then this can be hard to get used to at first. However, many breakfast skippers actually instinctively eat this way. You can drink <u>water</u>, <u>tea,</u> and other non-caloric beverages during the fast, and this can help reduce hunger levels. It is very important to eat mostly healthy foods during your eating window. This won't work if you eat lots of junk food or excessive amounts of calories.
   b. 20:4: This involves a 4-hour eating window and a 20-hour fast. For example, you might eat between 2:00 pm and 6:00 pm every day and

fast for the other 20 hours. Generally, this would involve eating either one meal or two smaller meals within this period.

2. Longer fasts (>24 hours)

    a. 24-hour fasts: This way of doing intermittent fasting involves fasting from dinner to dinner (or lunch to lunch). If you eat dinner on day 1, you would skip the next day's breakfast and lunch and eat dinner again on day 2. This means that you are still eating daily, but only once during that day. This would generally be done two to three times per week. Water, tea, and other non-caloric beverages are allowed during the fast, but no solid food.

    b. 5:2 fast: This involves 5 regular eating days and 2 fasting days. However, on these two fasting days, it is permitted to eat 500 – 600 calories on each day. These calories can be consumed at any time during the day – either spread throughout the day, or as a single meal. This diet is also called the Fast diet. On the fasting days, it is recommended that women eat 500 calories, and men 600 calories.

    c. 36-hour fasts: This involves fasting for the entire day. For example, if you eat dinner on day 1, you would fast for all of day 2 and not eat again until breakfast on day 3. This is generally 36 hours of fasting. This provides more powerful weight loss benefit. The other great benefit is that it avoids the temptation to overeat dinner on day 2.

3. Alternate-Day Fasting: Fast every other day. This is not recommended for beginners.

You should not intermittent fast if you are:

1. Underweight (Body Mass Index < 18.5)
2. Pregnant: you need extra nutrients for your child.
3. Breastfeeding: you need extra nutrients for your child.
4. A child under the age of 18: you need extra nutrients to grow.

You can fast, but you may require supervision, under the following conditions:

1.   If you have type 1 or type 2 diabetes mellitus
2.   If you currently take prescriptions
3.   If you have gout or high uric acid

You should continue all of your usual activities during fasting including exercise. If you exercise while you are fasting, your system will burn body fat for energy.

Tips for intermittent fasting:

1.   Drink water
2.   Stay busy
3.   Drink herbal tea
4.   Endure hunger waves
5.   Don't inform anyone who is not supportive
6.   Give yourself one month
7.   Follow a low-carb diet between fasting periods. This reduces hunger and makes fasting much easier. It may also increase the effect on weight loss and type 2 diabetes reversal, etc.
8.   Don't binge after fasting

How to get started:

Decide what type of fast you want to do

1.   Decide upon the length of time you want to fast

2.   Start fasting. If you do not feel well, or if you have any concerns, then stop and seek help

3.   Continue all your usual activities outside of eating. Stay busy and live normally. Imagine you're "eating" a full meal of your own fat

4.   Break the fast gently

5.   Repeat

If you experience nausea, dizziness, cramps, pain, or discomfort as you attempt to fast, please contact your primary doctor as soon as possible. If you have preexisting medical conditions, please consult your primary doctor prior to starting any fast.

Chapter 12

Limited Saturated Fat & Unlimited Saturated Fat

Some experts believe saturated fat tends to raise the level of <u>cholesterol</u> in the blood. Some experts believe saturated fat is a type of dietary fat and is one of the unhealthy fats, along with trans-fat. Foods like butter, palm and coconut oils, cheese, and red meat have high amounts of saturated fat. These experts believe too much saturated fat in your diet can lead to heart disease and other health problems. These experts believe your body needs healthy fats for energy and other functions. They believe too much saturated fat can cause cholesterol to build up in your arteries (blood vessels). Saturated fats raise your LDL (bad) cholesterol. They believe high LDL cholesterol increases your risk for heart disease and stroke.

Cholesterol and fats are both lipids and they are found both in the food you eat and circulating in your bloodstream. Cholesterol has a more complex chemical structure when compared to fats. In the body, cholesterol is bound to protein as low-density lipoprotein (LDL) which is considered to be the "bad cholesterol," for heart health risks, and high-density lipoprotein (HDL), which is called the "good cholesterol." Some experts believe the amount of unsaturated fat in your diet can influence your levels of total cholesterol, HDL, and LDL. Saturated fats have been said to raise LDL levels.

A saturated fat is a type of fat in which the fatty acid chains have all or predominantly single bonds. A fat is made of two kinds of smaller molecules: glycerol and fatty acids. Fats are made of long chains of carbon (C) atoms. Some carbon atoms are linked by single bonds (-C-C-) and others are linked by double bonds (-C=C-). Double bonds can react with hydrogen to form single bonds. They are called saturated, because the second bond is broken up and each half of the bond is attached to (saturated with) a hydrogen atom. Most animal fats are saturated. The fats of plants and fish are generally unsaturated. Saturated fats tend to have higher melting points than their corresponding unsaturated fats, leading to the popular understanding that saturated fats tend to be solids at room temperatures, while unsaturated fats tend to be liquid at room temperature with varying degrees of viscosity (meaning both saturated and unsaturated fats are found to be liquid at body temperature).

On the contrary, some experts believe differently about saturated fat. These experts believe saturated fat provides the following health benefits:

1. They believe saturated fat plays a couple of key roles in cardiovascular health. The addition of saturated fat to the diet reduces the levels of a substance called lipoprotein (a)—pronounced "lipoprotein little a" and abbreviated Lp(a)—that correlates strongly with risk for heart disease. Currently there are no medications to lower this substance and the only dietary means of lowering Lp(a) is eating saturated fat. These experts believe eating saturated (and other) fats also raises the level of HDL, the so-called good cholesterol. They reference research which has shown that when women diet, those eating the greatest percentage of the total fat in their diets as saturated fat lose the most weight.

2. They believe saturated fat intake can lead to weight loss. They believe that eating saturated fat does not make anyone fat. While you can technically overeat enough fat calories to accumulate adipose tissue, thus getting fat, this is a difficult feat, for two primary reasons:

   a. Fat is very satiating, especially when paired with low-carb eating. Grass-fed pot roast, ribbed with yellow fat, connective tissue, and ample protein is far more filling than some crusty bread spread with butter. You'll eat a decent slice of the former and be done, but you could easily polish off half a loaf of the latter with half a stick of butter and still be hungry. It's difficult to overeat on a high-fat, low-carb diet.

   b. Dietary fat in the presence of large amounts of dietary carbohydrates can make it difficult to access fat for energy, while dietary fat in the presence of low levels of dietary carbohydrates makes it easier to access fat for energy. Couple that with the fact that fat and carbs are easier to overeat together, and you have your explanation. In fact, studies have shown that low-carb, high-fat diets not only reduce weight, they also retain or even increase lean mass. That means it's fat that's being lost (rather than the nebulous "weight"), which is what we're ultimately after.

3. They believe eating saturated fat promotes liver health.

Adding saturated fat to the diet has been shown in medical research to encourage the liver cells to dump their fat content. Clearing fat from the liver is the critical first step to calling a halt to middle-body fat storage. Additionally, saturated fat has been shown to protect the liver from the toxic insults of alcohol and medications, including acetaminophen and other drugs commonly used for pain and arthritis, such as nonsteroidal anti-inflammatory drugs or NSAIDs, and even to reverse the damage once it has occurred. Since the liver is the lynchpin of a healthy metabolism, anything that is good for the liver is good for getting rid of fat in the middle. Polyunsaturated vegetable fats do not offer this protection.

2. They believe saturated fats improve brain function.

The brain is made largely of fat and the majority of the fat in the brain is saturated. The Myelin Sheath that surrounds the nerves in the brain and ensures their proper function is also largely made of saturated fat and cholesterol. As such, consuming saturated fats is extremely important, especially during pregnancy and nursing as these are times of rapid brain development for babies.

3. They believe eating saturated fats promotes healthier skin.

They argue the body needs healthy fats, including saturated fats, monounsaturated fats, and Omega-3 fats, to regenerate skin tissue, and these fats are the preferred building blocks in the body. If the body doesn't get these fats (and many people don't these days), it will use whatever it has available, including Omega-6 fats, which are not the preferred fat for building skin and collagen and can cause mutation (cancer).

6. They believe eating saturated fat promotes immune health.
    Saturated fats are also important for keeping the immune system
    functioning properly. Saturated fats found in butter, myristic acid, and
    lauric acid play key roles in immune health. Loss of sufficient saturated
    fatty acids in the white blood cells hampers their ability to recognize
    and destroy foreign invaders, such as viruses, bacteria, and fungi. Human
    breast milk is quite rich in myristic and lauric acid, which have potent
    germ-killing ability. But the importance of the fats lives on beyond
    infancy; we need dietary replenishment of them throughout adulthood,
    middle age, and into seniority to keep the immune system vigilant against
    the development of cancerous cells as well as infectious invaders.

According to the American Heart Association, your daily intake of
saturated fat should be approximately 13 grams per day. Experts suggest
substituting unsaturated fat for saturated fat. They suggest eating more
unsaturated fat and saturated fat.

Unsaturated fats are typically liquid at room temperature. They differ
from saturated fats in that their chemical structure contains one or more
double bonds.

Unsaturated fat can be categorized as:

1. Monounsaturated fats: This type of unsaturated fat contains only one
   double bond in its structure. Monounsaturated fatty acids, also known
   as omega-9 fatty acids, do a great deal to protect the heart.
   Monounsaturated fatty acids are associated with a slight yet significant
   effect on both systolic and diastolic blood pressure compared with a
   diet low in monounsaturated fatty acids. They also appear to improve
   insulin sensitivity when they replace either saturated fatty acids or
   carbohydrate in the diets of both healthy and insulin-resistant
   individuals. The effects of monounsaturated fatty acids on lipids vary.
   When monounsaturated fatty acids replace saturated fatty acids, LDL and
   total cholesterol drop by 6% to 10%. There's no effect on HDL
   cholesterol, although monounsaturated fatty acids favorably reduce the
   total cholesterol to HDL cholesterol ratio. Both HDL and triglyceride

levels improve, however, when monounsaturated fatty acids replace carbohydrate. Emerging research also suggests that monounsaturated fatty acids can cause a notable reduction in abdominal fat. In a study presented at the American Heart Association's (AHA) 2013 Scientific Sessions in New Orleans, subjects who consumed a daily smoothie high in monounsaturated fat for four weeks as part of a weight maintenance heart-healthy diet found their abdominal fat decreased by 1.6%. Abdominal fat was unchanged in those consuming a smoothie low in monounsaturated fats.

2. Polyunsaturated fats: This type of unsaturated fat contains two or more double bonds in their structure. They are liquid at room temperature. These are essential fatty acids that the body needs for brain function and cell growth. Polyunsaturated fatty acids include both omega-3 and omega-6 fatty acids. Some experts believe polyunsaturated fats decrease LDL and total cholesterol 8% to 12% when compared with saturated fatty acids. Consuming EPA and DHA, the long-chain omega-3 fatty acids found in cold-water fish, can improve blood triglyceride and HDL cholesterol levels. Alpha-linolenic acid (ALA), the short-chain omega-3 fatty acid found in some plants, as well as the two long-chain omega-3 fatty acids have beneficial effects on blood pressure and insulin sensitivity, she says. The America Heart Association recommends eating oily fish at least twice per week to obtain EPA and DHA and to regularly consume oils, walnuts, and other foods rich in ALA.5 Unfortunately, Americans consume, on average, one fish meal every 10 days, and it includes fish sticks and fried fish, which typically are low in omega-3 fats. Omega-3 fatty acids comprise only about 10% of total polyunsaturated fat intake. The majority of omega-3 intake comes from plant-sourced ALA, but Americans need more from EPA and DHA. Research shows that omega-6 fatty acids also may be cardioprotective. Some consumers and health professionals have expressed concern about consuming too much omega-6 fatty acids for fear of disrupting the omega-6 to omega-3 ratio, but many experts now say not to worry. Though it was once believed that omega-6 fatty acids increased arachidonic acid, the precursor to inflammatory compounds, researchers have found this isn't true. In 2009, the American Heart Association published a science advisory about omega-6 fatty acids and the risk of cardiovascular disease. It stated that although increasing omega-3 fats

reduces the risk of coronary heart disease (CHD), it doesn't follow that decreasing omega-6 fats will do the same. Researchers concluded that consuming 5% to 10% of calories from omega-6 fatty acids reduces CHD risk. Currently, Americans consume, on average, 7% of calories from omega-6 fatty acids. To recommend Americans lower their intake further would more likely increase rather than decrease CHD risk. Reinforcing this position is the report of the 2008 joint meeting of the Food and Agricultural Organization (FAO) of the United Nations and the World Health Organization (WHO) on fats and fatty acids on human health. The report concluded there's no rationale for a specific ratio of omega-6 to omega-3 fatty acids and that an appropriate intake of omega-6 fats is 2.5% to 9% of energy. Some experts believe omega-6 fatty acids slightly lower HDL cholesterol. Some experts believe the substantial improvement in total and LDL cholesterol more than offsets this effect, resulting in a favorable reduction in the total cholesterol to HDL cholesterol ratio compared with saturated fatty acids. Some experts still believe omega-6 fatty acids should be reduced because they compete with omega-3 fatty acids for the same enzymes, leading to the development of either proinflammatory or anti-inflammatory compounds. A recent reanalysis of the Sydney Diet Heart Study revealed that intakes of omega-6 fatty acids at 15% of energy resulted in an increase in the rates of death from all causes, coronary heart disease, and cardiovascular disease among men with a recent coronary event. Since current American intakes of omega-6 fatty acids are 7% of calories and within dietary guidelines, the focus should be on increasing omega-3 fatty acids, especially EPA and DHA, which would inevitably result in a decrease in the omega-6 to omega-3 ratio.

Omega 3-6-9 are polyunsaturated fatty acids, or healthy fats, that are important for human health. Of these fatty acids, omega 3 and omega 6 are referred to as essential fatty acids because they cannot be produced within the body and must be obtained through the diet. Omega 9 can be made in the body from other unsaturated fats consumed in the diet. Each of these omega fats has a slightly different side effect on the body, especially if you get too much.

Omega-3 is the most important of the omega fats, because it is more difficult to obtain in the diet and is less common in foods, when compared to omega-6 and omega-9. These fatty acids are found in fish foods and some plants and nuts. The main benefit of omega-3 is its anti-inflammatory qualities in terms of injury and excessive blood clotting. The University of Maryland Medical Center (UMMC) also recognizes omega-3 as being vital for proper brain function. If this fatty acid is being consumed by means of supplementation, it is not recommended to consume more than 3 g daily as there is a risk of excessive bleeding and increased sensitivity in bruising. Fish oil supplements of omega-3 are also known to cause bloating, belching and diarrhea in some cases.

Omega-3 fatty acids are good for your heart in several ways:

1. Reduce triglycerides, a type of fat in your blood

2. Reduce the risk of developing an irregular heartbeat (arrhythmia)

3. Slow the buildup of plaque in your arteries

4. Slightly lower your blood pressure

Omega-6 is similar to omega-3 in that it is also considered an essential fatty acid and that the body is unable to produce it from other unsaturated fats. Omega-6, however, is much easier to obtain through the diet. In fact, many people get too much omega-6 because it is found in so many common products, such as the butters and oils used in many cooking and baking processes in both home- and factory-prepared foods. Side effects of too much omega-6 cause an inflammatory reaction in the body. Although this is a desired side effect in some cases in terms of desired blood clotting when needed, over consumption can be harmful. According to the UMMC, evening primrose oil as an omega-6 supplement has side effects of headaches, abdominal pain, nausea and loose stools.

Omega-6 fatty acids may help:

1. Control your blood sugar

2. Reduce your risk for diabetes

3. Lower your blood pressure

Omega-9 fatty acid is not considered an essential fatty acid because the body can produce this substance on its own from other saturated fats consumed in the diet. The body can use omega-9 as a substitute for omega-3 and omega-6 if they are not present in the system. Omega-9 is found in animal fats, vegetable oils and cooking oils, such as olive oil. For omega-9 amounts to cause a problem, the intake would have to be associated with a diet that is very high in fat and dietary cholesterol, which is associated with weight gain and cardiovascular disease.

Fish oil can be obtained from eating fish or by taking supplements. Fish that are especially rich in the beneficial oils known as omega-3 fatty acids include mackerel, herring, tuna, salmon, cod liver, whale blubber, and seal blubber. Two of the most important omega-3 fatty acids contained in fish oil are eicosapentaenoic acid (EPA) and docosahexaenoic acid (DHA). Make sure to see separate listings on EPA and DHA, as well as Cod Liver Oil, and Shark Liver Oil. Fish oil is FDA approved to lower triglycerides levels, but it is also used for many other conditions. It is most often used for conditions related to the heart and blood system. Some people use fish oil to lower blood pressure, triglycerides and cholesterol levels. Fish oil has also been used for preventing heart disease or stroke, as well as for clogged arteries, chest pain, irregular heartbeat, bypass surgery, heart failure, rapid heartbeat, preventing blood clots, and high blood pressure after a heart transplant. Fish oil is also used to for many kidney-related problems including kidney disease, kidney failure, and kidney complications related to diabetes, cirrhosis, Berger's disease (IgA nephropathy), heart transplantation, or using the drug called cyclosporine.

Fish may have earned its reputation as "brain food" because some people eat fish to help with depression, bipolar disorder, psychosis, attention deficit-hyperactivity disorder (ADHD), Alzheimer's disease, developmental coordination disorder, migraine headache, epilepsy, schizophrenia, post-traumatic stress disorder, and mental impairment. Some people use fish oil for dry eyes, cataracts, glaucoma, and age-related macular degeneration (AMD), a very common condition in older people that can lead to serious sight problems. It is also used to prevent eye complications related to diabetes.

Fish oil is taken by mouth for stomach ulcers caused by Helicobacter pylori (H. pylori), inflammatory bowel disease, pancreatitis, an inherited disorder called phenylketonuria, allergy to salicylate, Crohn's disease, Behcet's syndrome, and Raynaud's syndrome.

Women sometimes take fish oil to prevent painful periods; breast pain; and complications associated with pregnancy such as miscarriage (including that caused by a condition called antiphospholipid syndrome), high blood pressure late in pregnancy, early delivery, slow infant growth, and to promote infant development.

Fish oil is also taken by mouth for weight loss, exercise performance and muscle strength, muscle soreness after exercise, pneumonia, cancer, lung disease, seasonal allergies, chronic fatigue syndrome, and for preventing blood vessels from re-narrowing after surgery to widen them.

Fish oil is also used for diabetes, prediabetes, asthma, a movement and coordination disorder called dyspraxia, dyslexia, eczema, autism, obesity, weak bones (osteoporosis), rheumatoid arthritis (RA), osteoarthritis, psoriasis, an autoimmune disease called systemic lupus erythematosus (SLE), multiple sclerosis, HIV/AIDS, cystic fibrosis, gum disease, Lyme disease, sickle cell disease, and preventing weight loss caused by some cancer drugs.

Fish oil is used intravenously (by IV) for scaly and itchy skin (psoriasis), blood infection, cystic fibrosis, pressure ulcers, and rheumatoid arthritis (RA). It is also used to prevent liver injury in people who are given food in the vein for long periods of time. Fish oil is applied to the skin for psoriasis.

A lot of the benefit of fish oil seems to come from the omega-3 fatty acids that it contains. Interestingly, the body does not produce its own omega-3 fatty acids. Nor can the body make omega-3 fatty acids from omega-6 fatty acids, which are common in the Western diet. A lot of research has been done on EPA and DHA, two types of omega-3 acids that are often included in fish oil supplements. Omega-3 fatty acids reduce pain and swelling. This may explain why fish oil is likely effective for psoriasis and dry eyes. These fatty acids also prevent the blood from clotting easily. This might explain why fish oil is helpful for some heart conditions.

Some experts recommend everyone take two to three grams daily of a fish oil supplement. They caution you to look for one derived from molecularly distilled fish oils, which are free of mercury, PCB, and other contaminants.

Some experts believe you cannot take too much omega-3s. There is, however, one exception, for individuals who take anti-coagulant drugs or have blood coagulation problems. They probably should avoid fish oil supplements since omega-3s can affect blood clotting. Very high intakes of fish oil/omega-3 fatty acids may increase the risk of hemorrhagic stroke and have been associated with nosebleed and blood in the urine.

Possible interactions involving fish oil include:

1. Anticoagulant and anti-platelet drugs, herbs and supplements: These types of drugs, herbs and supplements reduce blood clotting. It's possible that taking fish oil supplements with them might increase the risk of bleeding.

2. Blood pressure drugs, herbs, and supplements: Taking fish oil supplements might slightly lower blood pressure. Taking these supplements with blood pressure drugs might increase the effects on blood pressure.

3. Contraceptive drugs: Some contraceptive drugs might interfere with the effect fish oil typically has on triglycerides.

4. Orlistat (Xenical, Alli): Taking fish oil with this weight-loss drug might decrease absorption of fish oil fatty acids. Consider taking the supplement and drug two hours apart.

5. Vitamin E: Taking fish oil can reduce vitamin E levels.

The Weston A. Price Foundation reports that cod liver oil containing substantial levels of omega-3 EPA can actually contribute to hemorrhage during the birth process if not balanced by arachidonic acid (ARA), that equally important omega-6 fatty acid found in liver, egg yolks and meat fats. For this reason, pregnant women taking cod liver oil to benefit themselves and their baby must be sure to follow an entirely Traditional Diet during pregnancy and nursing and not just take cod liver oil as part of a nutrient poor, ARA deficient conventional diet. Some experts believe you should consume heart healthy omega-3 fats as part of a diet that also includes meat, liver and eggs.

Eating too much of any type of food or too many calories is never a good idea. Problems can arise if we eat too much fat — even healthy fat — since dietary fats have more than twice the calories per gram as proteins or carbohydrates. This is especially true if you couple the fat with sugars and processed carbs. It's not the fat itself but this combination that influences your metabolism by increasing inflammation, which could be the root of many chronic illnesses like heart disease, arthritis, diabetes, and cancer.

Side Effects of Too Much Fish Oil:

1. High Blood Sugar:

   Some research shows that supplementing with high amounts of omega-3 fatty acids could increase blood sugar levels in people with diabetes. This is because large doses of omega-3s can stimulate the production of glucose, which can contribute to high levels of long-term blood sugar levels. However, other research has turned up conflicting results, suggesting that only very high doses impact blood sugar. Another analysis of 20 studies found that daily doses of up to 3.9 grams of EPA and 3.7 grams of DHA — the two main forms of omega-3 fatty acids — had no effect on blood sugar levels for individuals with type 2 diabetes.

2. Bleeding

   Bleeding gums and nosebleeds are two of the side effects of excess fish oil consumption. One study in 56 people found that supplementing with 640 mg of fish oil per day over a four-week period decreased blood clotting in healthy adults. For this reason, it's often advised to stop taking fish oil prior to surgery and to talk to your doctor before taking supplements if you're on blood thinners like Warfarin.

3. Low Blood Pressure

Fish oil's capacity to lower blood pressure is well documented. While these effects can certainly be beneficial for those with high blood pressure, it can cause serious problems for those who have low blood pressure. Fish oil may also interact with blood pressure-lowering medications, so it's important to discuss supplements with your doctor if you're receiving treatment for high blood pressure.

4. Diarrhea

Diarrhea is one of the most common side effects associated with taking fish oil, and may be especially prevalent while taking high doses. In fact, one review reported that diarrhea is one of the most common adverse effects of fish oil, alongside other digestive symptoms such as flatulence. In addition to fish oil, other types of omega-3 supplements may also cause diarrhea. Flaxseed oil, for example, is a popular vegetarian alternative to fish oil, but has been shown to have a laxative effect and may increase bowel movement frequency. If you experience diarrhea after taking omega-3 fatty acids, make sure you're taking your supplements with meals and consider decreasing your dosage to see if symptoms persist.

5. Acid Reflux

Some people report feeling heartburn after starting to take fish oil supplements. Other acid reflux symptoms — including belching, nausea and stomach discomfort — are common side effects of fish oil due largely to its high fat content. Fat has been shown to trigger indigestion in several studies. Sticking to a moderate dose and taking supplements with meals can often effectively reduce acid reflux and relieve symptoms. Additionally, splitting your dose into a few smaller portions throughout the day may help eliminate indigestion.

6. Stroke

Hemorrhagic stroke is a condition characterized by bleeding in the brain, usually caused by the rupture of weakened blood vessels. Some animal studies have found that a high intake of omega-3 fatty acids could decrease the blood's ability to clot and increase the risk of hemorrhagic stroke. These findings are also consistent with other research showing that fish oil could inhibit blood clot formation. However, other studies have turned up mixed results, reporting that there is no association between fish and fish oil intake and hemorrhagic stroke risk. Further human studies should be conducted to determine how omega-3 fatty acids may impact the risk of hemorrhagic stroke.

7. Vitamin A Toxicity

Certain types of omega-3 fatty acid supplements are high in vitamin A, which can be toxic if consumed in large amounts. For example, just one tablespoon (14 grams) of cod liver oil can fulfill up to 270% of your daily vitamin A needs in one serving. Vitamin A toxicity can cause side effects such as dizziness, nausea, joint pain and skin irritation. Long term, it could also lead to liver damage and even liver failure in severe cases. For this reason, it's best to pay close attention to the vitamin A content of your omega-3 supplement and keep your dosage moderate.

8. Insomnia

In some cases, though, taking too much fish oil may actually interfere with sleep and contribute to insomnia. In one case study, it was reported that taking a high dose of fish oil worsened symptoms of insomnia and anxiety for a patient with a history of depression. However, current research is limited to case studies and anecdotal reports. More research is needed to understand how large doses may affect sleep quality in the general population.

Although recommendations can vary widely, most health organizations recommend an intake of at least 250-500 milligrams of combined

EPA and <u>DHA</u>, the two essential forms of omega-3 fatty acids, per day. However, a higher amount is often recommended for people with certain health conditions, such as heart disease or high triglyceride levels. For reference, a typical 1,000-mg fish oil soft gel generally contains about 250 mg of combined EPA and DHA, while one teaspoon (5 ml) of liquid fish oil packs in around 1,300 mg. According to the European Food Safety Authority, omega-3 fatty acid supplements can be safely consumed at doses up to 5,000 mg daily. As a general rule of thumb, if you experience any negative symptoms, simply decrease your intake or consider meeting your omega-3 fatty acid needs through <u>food sources</u> instead.

The American Heart Association recommends that most of your daily fat intake should come from monounsaturated and polyunsaturated fats. Foods containing unsaturated fats include:

1. Nuts

2. Certain fish like salmon, tuna, and anchovy, which contain omega-3 unsaturated fatty acids (Experts recommend eating fish at least twice weekly.)

3. Avocados

Some experts suggest you keep total fat consumption to no more than 25% to 30% of your daily calories. This includes monounsaturated and polyunsaturated fats. Eating healthier fats can lead to certain health benefits. But eating too much fat can lead to weight gain. All fats contain 9 calories per gram. This is more than twice the amount of calories found in carbohydrates and protein. It is not enough to add foods high in unsaturated fats to a diet filled with unhealthy foods and fats. Instead, replace saturated or trans-fats with healthier fats. Some experts believe eliminating saturated fats is twice as effective in lowering blood cholesterol levels as increasing polyunsaturated fats. They also strongly suggest your read nutrition labels to see the total fat in 1 serving.

Some experts believe the key is balancing your omega 3, 6, 9 ratio. One of the primary keys to good health is maintaining a proper omega 3 6 9 ratio of fatty acids in your diet. Researchers agree that the optimal omega ratio should be between 2:1 to 4:1. That is, you should consume at least double the amount of omega-3s compared to the other fats. Although soybean, corn, and canola oils are the omega-6 oils we should avoid, there are some healthy omega-6 fatty acids that do not cause inflammation and are actually good for the body. It isn't so much that one omega is inherently bad and another good; we just need an omega 3 6 9 ratio balance. The table below shows the healthy omega-3, omega-6, and omega-9 fatty acids that you should consume regularly as part of your healthy eating plan. Remember, you should try to consume at least a 2:1 omega 3 ratio over the other fats.

Healthy Omega Fatty Acid Sources:		
Omega-3s: Polyunsaturated (PUFA's)	Omega-6s: Polyunsaturated (PUFA's)	Omega-9s: Monounsaturated (MUFA's)
Cod liver oil	Borage oil (GLA)	Avocados
Flax seed & flax seed oil	Evening primrose oil (GLA)	Nuts (raw) - except peanuts
Fish oil	Egg Yolks	
Wild seafood	Animal Meats	
Walnuts		
Broccoli & cauliflower		
Spices (basil, oregano, cloves, marjoram)		

Trans-fat: An unhealthy substance, also known as trans fatty acid, made through the chemical process of hydrogenation of oils. Hydrogenation solidifies liquid oils and increases the shelf life and the flavor stability of oils and foods that contain them. Trans-fat is found in vegetable shortenings and in some margarines, crackers, cookies, snack foods and other foods. Trans-_fats_ are also found in abundance in French fries. Trans-fats can be found in many foods – including fried foods like doughnuts, and baked goods including cakes, pie crusts, biscuits, frozen pizza, cookies, crackers, and stick margarines and other spreads. You can determine the amount of trans-fats in a particular packaged food by looking at the Nutrition Facts panel. However, products can be listed as "0 grams of trans fats" if they contain 0 grams to less than 0.5 grams of trans-fat per serving. You can also spot trans-fats by reading ingredient lists and looking for the ingredients referred to as "partially hydrogenated oils". Small amounts of trans fats occur naturally in some meat and dairy products, including beef, lamb, and butterfat. There have not been sufficient studies to determine whether these naturally occurring trans-fats have the same bad effects on cholesterol levels as trans-fats that have been industrially manufactured. To make vegetable oils suitable for _deep_ frying, the oils are subjected to hydrogenation, which creates trans-fats. Among the hazards of fast food, "fries" are prime in purveying trans-fats.

Trans-fats wreak havoc with the body's ability to regulate _cholesterol_. In the hierarchy of fats, the polyunsaturated fats which are found in vegetables are the good kind; they lower your cholesterol. Saturated fats have been condemned as the bad kind. But trans-fats are far worse. They drive up the _LDL_ ("bad") cholesterol, which markedly increases the risk of coronary artery heart disease and _stroke_. According to a recent study of some 80,000 women, for every 5% increase in the amount of saturated _fat_ a woman consumes, her risk of heart disease increases by 17%. But only a 2% increase in trans-fats will increase her risk of heart disease

Chapter 13

Vegetables and Fruits

UPDATE:

I began consumption of raw (not juiced) vegetables and fruits. However, I believe there are numerous benefits to juiced organic vegetables and fruits.

The vast majority of modern weight loss programs do not heavily emphasize consumption of fresh vegetables and fruits. This was heavily emphasized back then. Some argue that modern vegetables and fruits are nutrient depleted due to nutrient depleted soil. In other words, vegetables and fruits today contain less nutritional value than the vegetables and fruit back then? Is this applicable to fresh organic vegetables and fruits? Limited research suggests depletion of nutrients within produce, which is why we should consume more vegetables and fruits. Fruits and veggies are still loaded with those all-important nutrients. Yet our soil is getting depleted and this is becoming a problem. This is another reason why you should consider purchasing organically grown vegetables and fruits.

Vegetables and fruits have dietetic value, nutritive value and some may also have the medicinal value. The dietetic value is a prophylactic (preventive) or curative quality of certain food stuffs and is natural. The main objective of the diet is the protection of the internal organs, first of those that participate directly or indirectly to digestion, of the blood-vascular system, etc. Fruits and vegetables have a natural dietetic importance because of their components like vitamin and minerals, dietary fibers, amino acids, Polyunsaturated Fatty Acids (PUFA) antioxidants and even phytoncides (natural antibiotics). The plant world particularly the group 'fruits and vegetables' is an enormous store of active chemical compounds and considered as the cheapest and most easily available sources of carbohydrate, fiber, proteins, vitamins, minerals and amino acids. The phytonutrients and nutraceuticals in fruits and vegetables are important. Vegetables and fruits offer medicinal and health benefits.

The term 'vegetable' includes any edible part of a plant. Vegetables are the cheapest and available sources of carbohydrates, proteins, vitamins and minerals. Leafy vegetables are said to be an invaluable substitute for meat and therefore form integral part of daily diets of rural communities. The traditional leafy vegetables have a proven nutritive value in terms of having high carbohydrate, protein, vitamins and minerals in comparison to that of exotic vegetables. Many of vegetables like carrot, radish, tomato, onion, cabbage and cucumber are routinely used as salad. There is growing trend of taking micro greens (seedlings of edible vegetables and herbs) for the sake of flavors, colors and textures and served as garnish or salad. Consumption of green salad is helpful in reducing the risk of chronic and cardiovascular disease. Consumption of low energy soup or vegetables before meal can reduce the intake of more energy dense food in children enhance satiety and control hunger and therefore helpful in managing weight. Swiss chard and salad crop have been reported to be rich in vitamins and minerals. The vitamin and mineral contents of peas is helpful in preventing diseases due to Selenium or folate deficiency.

Vegetables and fruits are packed with nutrients. We discussed nutrients in Chapter 7: Organic and Natural Supplements. Nutrients are the food substances that ensure normal deployment of biological and metabolic processes. The content of various nutrients is not as important as the quality, availability and ratio of the compounds. Many phytochemicals have been identified helping the body in maintenance of health and fighting various diseases. The term nutraceutical describes particular chemical compounds found in foods that may prevent disease development and phytochemical can underestimate the plant source of most of these protective compounds, whereas phytonutrient describes quasi-nutrient status of such compounds. The phytonutrients present in fruits and vegetables have been classified in the older times into vitamins, for example flavonoids were recognized as vitamin P, cabbage factors (glucosinolates and indoles) as vitamin U, ubiquinone as vitamin Q and Tocopherol as vitamin E. The phytonutrients can be classified into various groups on the basis of alike protective functions as well as individual physical and chemical characteristics of the molecules. It is important to note that all classes of phytonutrients are required to be consumed for a sound and healthy body.

Phytonutrients and their useful medicinal values:

1.   Anthocyanidins: Anthocyanidins are a type of flavonoids, also known as flavonols, which provide cross-links that hook up and strengthen the intertwined collagen protein strands found in tissues, tendons, ligaments and bone matrix. These also act as free radical scavenger in tissue fluids. In human beings, risk of myocardial infarction is reduced by taking high number of anthocyanins.

2.   Carotenoids: The carotenoid family consists of carotenes and xantophylls. There are more than 600 naturally occurring carotenoids. The subclass terpenes comprise of bright red, orange and yellow pigments present in various vegetables viz., tomatoes, spinach, oranges, pink grapefruit and red palm oil. Carotenes are chemically classified as 40-carbon tetraterpenes, missing the hydroxyl or keto groups (beta carotene), while xanthophylls include carotenoid alcohols and keto-carotenoids cryptoxanthin, canthaxanthin, zeaxanthin and astaxanthin. Vitamin A activity is only present in alpha, beta and epsilon carotene, out of these the beta carotene is the most active. The antioxidant activity of alpha carotene and epsilon carotene is 50-54 and 42-50%, respectively of the antioxidant activity of beta carotene. The alpha, beta, gamma, epsilon, lycopene and lutein carotenes have been found to be provide protection against tumors of the lung, colorectal, breast, uterine and prostate. The overall protective effects of carotenes will be additive if taken together, since the these are tissue-specific. The carotenes also augment immune response and can protect skin cells against UV radiation. These also help liver in safely eliminating pollutants and toxins from the body. Xanthophylls help in the protection of vitamin A, E and various other carotenoids from oxidation. Xanthophylls especially canthaxanthin migrates to the skin and protects

it from sunlight. The cryptoxanthin has been shown to protect vaginal, uterine and cervical tissues.

3.   Catechins, gallic acids: The chemical structure of catechins is slightly different from other flavonoids but has the same chemoprotective activities. Green tea (Camellia sinensis) is rich in catechins.

4.   Flavonoids: Flavonoids constitute a subclass of phenols that improve the effects of ascorbate-vitamin C. The hesperidin found in citrus fruits and quercetin in grapefruit are some of the most important flavonoids. These are beneficial in allergic conditions, inflammation, liver disorders, platelet aggregation, pathogens (bacteria and viruses), cancer and ulcers and acts as antioxidant. These inhibit a number of specific enzymes thereby help in preventing various diseases and maintenance of a healthy body. The flavonoids block the Angiotensin-converting Enzyme (ACE) that is responsible for raising blood pressure. The platelet stickiness and aggregation are prevented by blocking the cyclooxygenase enzyme that breaks down prostaglandins. Flavonoids are also helpful in protection of the vascular system. The risk of estrogen-induced cancers in females can be reduced by flavonoids due to blocking of certain enzymes producing estrogen. Aldose-reductase can convert the galactose sugar into the potentially harmful form of galacticol. Flavonoids may retard development of cataracts in individuals with inborn errors in sugar metabolism such as diabetes by blocking aldose-reductase.

5.   Glucosinolates: These are frequently present in the vegetables of *Cruciferi* family and set in motion the detoxification enzymes in liver, white blood cells and cytokines thereby helping in boosting immunity. The isothiocyanates, dithiolthiones and sulforaphane are the bio-transformation products of glucosinolates that are involved in blocking enzymes which are responsible for tumorous growth in liver, lung, breast and gastrointestinal tracts (esophagus, stomach and colon).

6.   Indoles: Indoles include phytonutrients that interact with vitamin C and their complexes bind with chemical carcinogens. These also help in activating the detoxification enzymes. The acid in stomach helps in the formation of bio-transformation products of indoles like the ascorbigen.

7.   Isoflavones: This is a subclass of phenol found in beans and other legumes and its function is similar to flavonoids in effectively block enzymes promoting tumor growth. Some experts believe the incidence of breast, uterine and prostate cancers is rare in people who consume traditional diets rich in soy foods.

8.   Isoprenoids: The isoprenoids neutralize free radicals by grabbing any free radicals attempting to attach lipid (fat) membranes passing them off to other antioxidants.

9.   Limonoids: This is a subclass of terpenes that is found in citrus fruit, a peel that is specifically directed to protect lung tissue and prevent breast cancer that responses to estrogen. The chemotherapeutic activity of limonoids may be due to induction of both Phase I and Phase II detoxification enzymes in the liver.

10.   Lipoic acid and ubiquinone: Lipoic acid and ubiquinone (coenzyme Q) are antioxidants which can efficiently quench the hydroxyl radicals and are active on both lipids and tissue fluids and scavenges peroxyl, ascorbyl and chromanoxyl radicals. It can protect both vitamin E and vitamin C, as can function in both lipid and water phases. They can also protect catalase and glutathione, thus helpful in liver detoxification activities.

11.   Phytosterols: Phytosterols are present in green and yellow vegetables and their seeds. These can effectively compete with dietary cholesterol absorption through intestines and thus make easy the excretion of cholesterol from the body and therefore are helpful in alleviating the risk of cardiovascular diseases. These have also been reported to be helpful in blocking the development of cancer in various organs especially colon, breast and prostate glands.

12.   Phenols: Phenols are a large group of phytonutrients protecting the humans from various kinds of oxidative damages. Phenol gives the blue, blue-red and violet colorations to berries, grapes and purple eggplant. The red color in bilberries is due to the presence of high phenolic anthocyanidins. The phenols block specific enzymes that cause inflammation and protect platelets from clumping most likely by modification of the prostaglandin pathways.

13.   Terpenes: These form the largest classes of phytonutrients and are commonly present in green foods, soy products and grains. Carotenoid i.e., beta carotene is one of the most studied terpenes. The antioxidants property of the terpenes protects lipids, blood and other body fluids from attack by free radical oxygen.

14.   Thiols: Thiols comprises of sulfur-containing phytonutrients present in garlic and cruciferous vegetables (cabbage, turnips and members of the mustard family). Allylic Sulfides subclass is abundantly found in garlic, onions, leeks, shallots and chives and are released when the plants are cut or smashed. These possess antimutagenic and anticarcinogenic properties as well as immune enhancing and cardiovascular protective properties. Garlic and onions activate liver detoxification enzyme systems and are also effective against tumors, bacteria, fungi, viruses, parasites, cholesterol and platelet/leukocyte adhesion factors.

15.   Tocotrienols and tocopherols: Tocotrienols and tocopherols naturally occur in grains and palm oil. Tocotrienols can suppress cancer cell growth but not the tocopherols, which on the other hand show cholesterol lowering effects.

One of the more unique things about vegetables is the belief that some vegetables act as medicines and are reserved for the sick and convalescence individuals because of their multi-dimensional medicinal properties. Nearly half the medicines being used today are of herbal origin and a quarter contains plant extracts or active chemicals taken directly from various plants. Many more have yet to be discovered as well as recorded and researched. Only a few thousand have been studied so far, carrot being a wonderful example. Carrot is a common vegetable that finds its way to the dining table in the salad as well as cooked greens. As a fruit, it is an excellent promoter of reproductive potential of man and animals but its seeds have proven anti-fertility role. The beta carotene and other carotenoids in carrot also provide protection against the oxidant induced changes in lipid peroxidation, deoxy glucose transport, LDH release and amino acid and also protect the skin from damaging effects of sunlight.

The medicinal value is subordinated to the nutraceutical value, may have medicinal properties, and can be administered as a therapeutic agent. Some vegetable foods have been recognized as natural medicines. Folate present in fresh leafy green vegetables is helpful in reducing the risk of chronic diseases that include: megaloblastic anemia; neural tube defects, cardiovascular disease and cancers.

The medicinal uses of various common vegetables range from burn ointments to diuretics. Parts of vegetables may be used to produce drugs, or may be an effective dietetic food. The lycopene present in tomato when present in the bloodstream has been shown to protect against oxidation of low-density lipoproteins and thus reduces the incidence of arterial disease. Epidemiological studies have also shown tomato consumption to reduce the risk of prostate cancer. The seeds of the carrot are reported to possess emmenagogue and abortifacient properties and are also used in uterine pain. Seeds of the pea (*Pisum sativum* L.) are reported to possess antifertility and abortifacient actions. Oil obtained from pea seeds have been found to elicit contraceptive action in albino rats. The active ingredient is m-xylohydroquinone; a single dose of 1 mg caused abortion, reabsorption, or still births in mice and rats. *Foeniculum* seeds are effective against hernias and hydrocele when used with other salts or ingredients. Radish and green chilies, a common constituent of salad, are good potentiators of uterine involution.

Vegetables can provide phytonutrients as well as nutritional components, such as vitamins, minerals and fiber. Some of dark green leafy vegetables like arugula, broccoli, spinach, kale and cabbage; dandelion greens; swiss chard and watercress etc., provide a variety of nutrients like vitamin A and B complex, vitamin E, major minerals (calcium and phosphorous) and trace minerals (manganese and potassium) etc. Root vegetables like beets are rich in vitamin B complex, vitamin C, manganese, magnesium, iron, copper and phosphorus. A close relative of Indian drumstick, Moringa stenopetala has highly nutritious leaves, edible flowers, edible pods, antibiotic properties in seeds and the bark is used as a hot condiment with one of the highest calcium levels and highest vitamin C levels. Young plantain leaves, consumed raw in salad in Asia, are rich source in vitamin B1 and riboflavin. Plantain are rich in various glycosides like aucubin, ascorbic acid, apigenin, baicalein, benzoic and chlorogenic acid; citric and ferulic acid; oleanolic and salicylic acid and ursolic acid, which are all having tremendous medicinal activities viz., antimicrobial, anti-inflammatory, antitussive, cardiac stimulant, diuretic, laxative, antitussive, antiseptic, poultice, refrigerant and vermifuge. The use of these drugs for the treatment of respiratory problems (asthma, bronchitis and emphysema), bladder disorders, pyrexia, cardio-vascular disorders (hypertension), rheumatism and blood sugar control has been scientifically proven. It also causes a natural aversion to tobacco and is currently being used in preventing smoking.

Vegetables are an amazing source of antioxidants and vitamins (β-carotene, vitamins C and E). Pumpkin, tomato, carrot, garlic, clove; the list is everlasting. Vegetables like carrots, pumpkins, acorn squash butternut squash, Hubbard squash and sweet potatoes, also known as orange vegetables, are a rich source of carotenoids, which act are known antioxidants. Due to presence of antioxidants, higher intake of green leafy vegetables and cruciferous vegetables reduces homocysteine and markers of oxidative stress thus leading to lower risk of bladder cancer, non-Hodgkin's lymphoma (NHL) and particularly follicular lymphoma. Increased consumption of vegetables has also been found to improve the Pneumovax II vaccination antibody response in older people, leading to improved immunity. Garlic clove is also well recognized for protection against bowel cancer. These antioxidants are also helpful in combating the oxidative stress induced by the environmental pollutants such as heavy metals and pesticides.

Out of more than 600 carotenoids present in plants, only few like alpha carotene, beta carotene, lycopene, zeaxanthin, lutein and betacryptoxanthine are utilized by human beings. The high level of α-carotene, β-carotene, lutein, zeaxanthin, lycopene and total carotenoids in blood circulation is helpful in reduced risk of breast cancer in women. Phytoene and phytofluene, precursors of higher unsaturated carotenoids are responsible for photoprotective effects. A USDA study also detected compromised immune function in otherwise healthy females fed on low carotene diet. Green leafy vegetables are rich in iron content required for synthesis of hemoglobin, hence suggested in iron deficiency anemia. Various minerals including the trace minerals are also co-enzymes in certain biochemical reactions in the body, which adds to the importance of leafy vegetables in metabolic reactions.

The fiber content of vegetables provides a bulk in the diet. This helps to reduce the intake of starchy foods, enhances gastrointestinal function, prevents constipation and may thus reduce the incidence of metabolic diseases like maturity onset, diabetes mellitus and hypercholesterolemia. The fiber cleanses the gut by removing the various carcinogens from the body and prevents the absorption of excess cholesterol. It also prevents the intake of excess starchy food and therefore protect against metabolic disorders (hypercholesterolemia and diabetes mellitus). Fiber from the seed coat and the cell walls of the cotyledon of peas is beneficial for gastrointestinal function and health.

Some vegetables are also potent antibiotics, antihypertensive and blood building agents and also improve fertility in females when eaten in soups. The phytochemical contents of the leafy vegetables provide nutritive supplements for food and also improve the health status of its consumers due to the existence of several compounds' fundamental for good health. Phytochemicals like polyphenolics and saponins present in colored seed coat of peas have potent antioxidant and anticarcinogenic properties. Polyphenols play critical role in prevention of various diseases including of cardiovascular, neurodegenerative disorders, diabetes mellitus, osteoporosis and even cancer, hepatic damage, inhibit angiogenesis and obesity. It is well known and proven fact that certain foods possess potential to effectively prevent many diseases as universal medicines. Consumption of green tea is beneficial for preventing cancer and Alzheimer's disease (AD). Green and yellow vegetables decrease the risk of chronic disease and inhibits the development of atherosclerosis. Therefore, it may lead to a reduction in the risk of coronary heart disease, stroke, markers of inflammation and oxidative stress, serum homocysteine and markers of protein, lipid and DNA oxidation. Such consumptions could also mitigate contaminant exposure and/or their adverse health effects. The presence of mucilage in some vegetables makes their soups tastier and more palatable.

Vegetables help in retaining stronger bones by decreasing the amount of calcium excreted in the urine. They also act as an alkaline buffer neutralizing acid produced when non-vegetarian diet is consumed. Major mineral components of the leaves include calcium, potassium, sodium, and iron. Calcium is a major component giving strong bones, muscle contraction and relaxation, synaptic transmission, blood clotting and absorption of Vitamin especially B_{12}. The relatively high content of calcium in Gryllotalpa Africana, potassium and magnesium are known to decrease blood pressure. Potassium plays a crucial role in skeletal muscle contraction and transmission of nerve impulses. Therefore, the persons having the soft bone are usually advised to have the vegetables rich in calcium and potassium.

Phytoconstituents of vegetables are also very effective stimulants for the nervous system of the body. The bitter leaf contains an alkaloid, vernomine, which is capable of reducing headaches associated with hypertension. Broccoli is as excellent source of sulforaphane, which has a powerful anti-cancerous effect. Spinach retards central nervous system and cognitive behavioral deficits. Ocimum species are rich in alkaloids that are useful in cold, cough, chronic catarrh and migraine. The medicinal importance of tannins, saponins and inulins which are components of traditional herbal preparations are highly useful in managing various common ailments. Lesser medication and more natural foods need to have a priority place in our life but to get maximum health benefits sufficient knowledge and understanding a necessity. The demarcation between nutritious/medicinal vegetables and toxic vegetables is very thin. The most commonly consumed tuber, potato (Solanum tuberosum), also contains a toxin, solanine which is destroyed by heat.

Freezing can slightly alter the nutritional composition of fruits and vegetables, sometimes in favor of the frozen product and sometimes in favor of the fresh. Though vitamins can degrade in fresh fruits and vegetables over time, many nutrients in foods are much harder than most people assume. Minerals like iron are almost bulletproof, and the fiber doesn't care at all whether it's heated or frozen. And in general, the differences in nutrient levels between fresh and frozen are so minor that they would be unlikely to have an impact on overall health.

Vitamin content was compared for eight different fresh and frozen fruits and vegetables — corn, carrots, broccoli, spinach, peas, green beans, strawberries and blueberries — and found no consistent differences over all between fresh and frozen. The vitamin content was occasionally higher in some frozen foods; frozen broccoli, for example, had more riboflavin (a B vitamin) than fresh broccoli. But frozen peas had less riboflavin than fresh peas; and frozen corn, green beans and blueberries had more vitamin C than their fresh counterparts. The researchers also analyzed the amount of fiber, levels of phenolic compounds (good sources of antioxidants) and minerals like calcium, iron, zinc and magnesium in the same eight fruits and vegetables. They found no significant differences between the fresh and frozen varieties. Fresh berries can lose some nutrients while sitting on the shelf, so eat them right away to get the most nutrients. Frozen berries will also deteriorate when kept in a home freezer that's opened and shut often. Freeze fruits in a deep freezer or at the very back of a kitchen freezer. Look for produce frozen under a process called "individually quick frozen," or IQF, for the best quality.

Canned and frozen versions are the most common processed vegetables. While processed vegetables can be more convenient, have a longer shelf-life, and are free from microorganisms that may cause disease, there's the potential that the nutritional quality of these foods is diminished. While many people feel that fresh veggies are optimal, they may lose nutrients before consumption. Because it could take up to two weeks from the time they've been picked until they're eaten, it's possible that 10 to 50 percent of the less stable nutrients have disappeared. Still, raw, lightly prepared, or minimally processed veggies (and fruits) often have a higher nutrient value than well-cooked ones.

To help preserve the nutrient content of veggies (and fruits) during cooking or other preparation:

1. Stick with shorter cooking times and lower temperatures (e.g., avoid deep frying).

2. Cook with little or no water to help retain water-soluble vitamins, such as vitamin C and the B vitamins. You might try steaming or

microwaving rather than boiling. To limit exposure to heat when cooking this way, wait until the water is boiling before adding veggies.

In terms of frozen and canned vegetables, they're often processed shortly after they're picked in order to minimize nutrient loss during shipping, on the grocer's shelf, or at home. Like frozen vegetables, canned ones are also processed right after being harvested. Most of the change in nutrition that occurs in frozen and canned vegetables is due to blanching. This process involves heating the veggies quickly with water or steam. The water-soluble vitamins, including vitamins B and C can be destroyed during this process. Sometimes, instead of high heat, food processing uses high pressures to kill microorganisms that may cause illness, which may preserve the nutrient quality, color, and taste of veggies better than other methods. Another form of veggie processing is dehydration. On one hand, this process can make fiber more concentrated, leading to better digestive regulation. On the other hand, dehydrated veggies may not retain the same amounts of vitamin C, and they're more energy dense than fresh foods (more calories in less food), which may lead to weight gain if not eaten in moderation. For example, sun-dried tomatoes are more calorie dense than raw tomatoes.

However, some experts believe fresh fruits and vegetables are better for you than canned or frozen, because the processing removes all of the nutrients.

Washing fruits and vegetables is very important. Contaminated vegetables and fruits can also make you sick. Add to that less-than-hygienic conditions during harvesting, packing, and transportation, and it becomes all too clear how fruits and vegetables get contaminated. More importantly, eating raw unwashed vegetables and fruits can cause internal parasites.

Vegetables and fruit washing tips:

1. Wash your hands properly.

   Wash your hands with lukewarm water and soap before handling any fresh fruit and vegetables. Or you could easily transfer MORE germs to your salad, instead of cleaning it.

2. Rinse fruits and vegetables under cold water.

   This helps in scrubbing off any remnants of soil clinging to it. This is particularly important for all root vegetables. Even if you are going to peel them before cooking, make sure you rinse them thoroughly. Or else your knife/peeler will pass on contaminants on the skin to the vegetable itself.

3. Be mindful of fresh whole vegetables.

   Washing fresh whole vegetables thoroughly is very important as these may have more soil and pesticides clinging to them compared to pre-cut vegetables. A good rinse with cold water and rubbing the skin underwater will remove most pesticides and bacteria from the skin, even E. coli.

4. Leafy green vegetables need special attention.

   All leafy green vegetables like spinach, cabbage, mustard, chard, and lettuce need special attention. The best way to clean lettuce or cabbage thoroughly is to remove the central core and outer leaves that have wilted. Separate the leaves and then clean them thoroughly by soaking them in a large bowl of water for 2-5 minutes. For spinach, mustard greens and arugula, soak and swirl them in the large bowl of water. This removes dirt hiding in between the leaves. Give the leaves a gentle rub, and then lift the leaves out of the water, give them a gentle shake, and put into the colander or salad spinner. Don't overturn the bowl of dirty water directly into the colander, as larger chunks of dirt and debris may still be caught in between your salad leaves.

5. Cut cruciferous vegetables and soak them.

Vegetables like cauliflower and broccoli should be cut, and then soaked in water for few minutes, as dust, grime and pesticides can be hiding in the nooks and crannies.

6. Certain fruits and vegetables need more thorough cleaning.

Some fruits and vegetables need a more thorough clean as they are very susceptible to mold, and hence sprayed extensively with pesticides. These include plums, grapes, berries, apples, peaches, pears, okra and eggplant. Wash them thoroughly in cold, clean, running water before eating them.

7. Don't soak mushrooms and berries.

Mushrooms and berries need a good rinse to clean them but shouldn't be soaked in water. Mushrooms, in particular, can spoil very quickly when they are soaked. Instead, hold mushrooms under cold, running water and gently rub to remove all dirt, grime and pesticides off the skin. Cooking the mushrooms will take care of any lurking bacteria. Both mushrooms and berries, like strawberries, are best washed right before eating. Once they have been exposed to water, they spoil rather quickly, so wash only as much as you will consume immediately.

8. Use clean towels for drying vegetables.

Once washed, make sure you dry all fruit and vegetable with clean kitchen towels. It's always a good idea to wash just before eating or cooking, as storing washed vegetables and fruits in the fridge can make them spoil faster.

9. Try a salt solution.

This is one of the easiest ways to kill germs sticking to fresh fruits and vegetables. This simple step can remove most of the contact pesticide residues, which normally linger on the surface of vegetables and fruits. Full up a bowl or your kitchen sink with clean water and add a teaspoon of salt. Now allow your fresh fruit or vegetable to soak in this salt solution for few minutes. If you want to clean salad greens effectively, you can add a squeeze of lime with the salt to the water to draw out all dirt, bacteria and pesticides. Now drain well and rinse with cold fresh water for a minute or so before using in any recipe.

10. Try a vinegar bath for fruits with a glossy coating.

Fruits and vegetables with a glossy coating may help preserve them for longer, but this wax coating also seals the contaminants within the fruit or vegetable. Think apples, pears, eggplant and grapes. This means that mere washing with water will not remove all germs in such fresh produce. By cleaning with a vinegar-water solution, the acidic medium will effectively remove wax and bacteria and give your fresh produce a thorough clean. You can add 1 part vinegar to 3 parts water and soak your fruit or vegetables in this solution for few minutes. Or you can mix vinegar and water in the same ratio in a spray bottle and spray generously over the fruit and vegetable. Allow to stand for 20-30 minutes, and then rinse thoroughly before eating.

11. Use a potassium permanganate solution.

We saved the best for last! A very diluted solution of potassium permanganate will effectively remove any pests, bacteria, parasites, worms and pesticide residue from fruits and vegetables, making them safer to eat. Washing fruits and vegetables with a solution of potassium permanganate can greatly help in controlling food-borne disease outbreak. Mix just a couple crystals of potassium permanganate in a liter of water so that the solution is just lightly tinted pink. If your solution is dark pink, you've added too many potassium permanganate crystals and need to dilute the solution further with water. Soak vegetables and fruits in this solution for 5 to 8 minutes. Then remove and rinse very well with cold running water.

In Chapter 6: Natural then Mostly Organic, we discussed the dangers of ingredients found in conventional household cleaning products. With this being said, why would anyone utilize conventional dish detergent to wash edible fresh vegetables and fruits? I purchase natural or organic fruit and vegetable washes to wash vegetables and fruits. I make sure I follow the directions very carefully. There are different directions for different brands. If the directions say to let it soak, you should allow the vegetables and fruits to soak. Even after I wash my carrots, I still carve off the outer skin and rewash just to make sure they are clean.

I make a conscientious effort to utilize my nutribullet daily to juice my vegetables and fruits. There are different types of nutribullet machines for different prices. The Nutribullet RX allows you to juice more at once than the 2 for 1 special. If you juice more than the nutribullet machine will allow you to at once, it will cut off. You won't be able to use the machine until the next day even if you have plugged the cord in an outlet. The Nutribullet RX allows you to juice a 14" x 20" tray of vegetables and fruits without cutting off. However, this should work if you cut your vegetables and fruits into smaller pieces and you don't leave the container filled with water, vegetables, and fruit in the machine too long.

I initially wanted a Vitamix machine, which is what Whole Foods utilize to make their smoothies. However, the Vitamix company did not offer any monthly payment plans at the time. I decided not to postpone this health endeavor due to an inability to afford the vitamix machine upfront. I decided to get the nutribullet machine. I initially made a small down payment then 6 subsequent $19.99 monthly payments for the 2-for-1 special that was offered on their website at the time.

The USDA (United States of Department of Agriculture currently recommends 5 to 13 servings of vegetables and fruits per day.

Serving sizes for vegetables:

1. One cup of a raw leafy vegetable is considered 1 serving.
2. One-half cup of fresh, frozen, or a canned vegetable is considered 1 serving.
3. One-half cup of vegetable juice is considered 1 serving.

Serving sizes for fruits:

1. One medium fruit is equivalent to 1 serving.
2. A half cup of fresh, frozen, or canned fruit is considered 1 serving.
3. One-fourth (1/4) cup of dried fruit is considered 1 serving.
4. A half cup of juice is considered 1 serving.

I tend to utilize my nutribullet differently. I do not make smoothies or juices solely for taste. The juice I make are solely for nutritional purposes. I include only fresh vegetables and fruits. I do not include frozen, canned, or steamed vegetables or fruits. I typically include organic: kale, broccoli, carrots, tomato, lemon, lime, blueberries, avocado, and water. As much as possible, I try to make sure I juice at least a combination of kale, avocado, broccoli, blueberries, and blackberries. I don't include a bunch of sugary fruits. If you do so, you are defeating the purpose. I only utilize water. No other beverages. I do not utilize tap water. This way I am getting my daily recommended amount of water intake and vegetable and fruit intake simultaneously. As a general rule of thumb, you are supposed to drink at least half of your body weight and no more than your entire body weigh in ounces of water on a daily basis. Factors such as activity level and whether or not you live in a warmer or cooler climate also may require you to drink more or less water.

I use bottled water at room temperature. I wash my vegetables and fruits off with organic or natural fruits and vegetable wash according to the instructions. I then cut up all of the above vegetables and fruits into smaller pieces with the exception of the blueberries. I only remove the exterior skin from the carrots, lemon, and lime. All of the above vegetables and fruits are cut into smaller pieces on a tray with the exception of blueberries, which have not been cut. The reason I utilize a tray is because I also juice for others. This is really why you should spend the extra bucks to purchase a Nutribullet RX, but I you are not currently able to do so. Start where you are at.

I then take and crush my multi-vitamin tablet into powder form. I also blend differently. I take the above vegetables and fruits that have been cut into smaller pieces and the place them within the larger container. I fill this container to the brim with these vegetables, fruits, and water. I blend this mixture for less than 5 seconds. I pour out a little more than half of this mixture into 1 of the smaller nutribullet RX containers. I pour my crushed multi-vitamin tablet powder on top of the mixture left in the larger container. I also add organic ground turmeric powder. Yes, you can add liquid or powder supplements to your nutribullet juice. However, you want to make sure you do not add to many different supplements at once. This can possibly make you nauseous.

I tend to drink my juice after my breakfast, because I make my juices early in the morning. Some experts recommend consuming these types of juices following meals, because these juices contain enzymes that will benefit the digestive process. I am a not aware of any experts who advise juicing on an empty stomach.

Then I blend (for a lack of a better word). Unless I have a conflicting work schedule or I have to utilize my Nutribullet RX before 6:00 a.m., I tend to drink the portion with the crushed multi-vitamin and turmeric powder immediately. This portion tends to be between 10 and 17.5 ounces. I then blend the other portion. I continue this pattern of filling the larger container to the brim with water, partially blending the larger container for a few seconds, pour out half or more of the mixture, and then I re-blend each portion until it has the texture of a juice. The reblending tends to also take less than 5 seconds with the Nutribullet RX unless there is too much mixture in the container.

When people tend to utilize the Nutribullet RX or a similar type of machine, they tend to juice or blend for several days at a time as opposed to what they are going to consume that very day. They pour their juices into smaller water bottles. This is not advised. The nutribullet is not a blender, but rather a food extractor. Extraction of vegetables and fruits while in the nutribullet can result in decreased nutrients and anti-oxidants. However, some experts disagree. These experts believe the nutrients and fiber within vegetables and fruits prior to extraction remains intact during extraction within the nutribullet. For this very reason, it is recommended to drink the juice either immediately or as soon as possible. Only juice enough for the day. I typically tend to finish juicing early in the morning, typically early morning hours. I typically finish most of the juice before the afternoon. Then I finish the rest of the juice before 6:00 p.m. Then I juice the next day. Whatever amount of unconsumed juice is left is discarded, not refrigerated. If you do otherwise, it is waste of vegetables, fruits, time, effort, and money.

I really encourage you to get a Nutribullet machine so you can get started as soon as possible. Some experts believe that since vegetables and fruits are in a liquified form, they can be digested faster. The stomach has sensory capabilities that help determine the nutritional content of what it receives. When the stomach receives traditional foods like carbohydrates, fats, and proteins, it adds protein-digesting enzymes such as pepsin and hydrochloric acid (HCL) to break down the nutrients for absorption in the intestines. The more complex the food, the longer it stays in the stomach. So protein can take hours. Liquids like tea, juice tend to be even less complicated, water least of all- taking possibly just minutes to start passing into the blood stream if there is no food in the stomach and fully entering the blood stream within 1-2 hours.

I was told by a dental student at a school to at least floss and goggle with mouthwash or floss and brush my teeth after I finished drinking my vegetable and fruit juice. I was advised that vegetable and fruit juice can cause acid erosion of your teeth. However, you have to consider all of the other health benefits.

The reason why I make juices instead of smoothies is because I still eat regular food. I drink my nutribullet juices in conjunction with eating food.

I do not solely drink only vegetable and fruit juice, but not eat food. I try to get my protein and fiber from the foods I eat. I typically consume organic cashews, organic uncooked cheese, organic plain yogurt with stevia added (without all of the added sugars), and other organic foods for my source of protein. I think these maybe considered nutrient dense foods. This would be okay if this was for a temporary juice detox fast, but not on a longer-term basis. Your body needs protein, fiber, etc.

When asked by others if I feel a difference internally as a result of my nutritional practices, especially Nutribullet juices, my response has been, "I feel the difference, because I am consistent in all areas. In essence, not just drinking the nutribullet vegetable and fruit juice then eating whatever whenever. Yes, you do feel a difference internally.

I personally think the nutribullet and similar machines are amazing. I want to thank whoever invented this machine. I believe it was Colin Sapire. This machine allows people to conveniently get the daily recommended amount of vegetables and fruits. You can also make soups with the nutribullet. You can even make meals for 6-month olds. You can cut up small chunks of cooked or preferably baked chicken, add a small scoop of mashed potatoes with gravy, cut up small pieces of carrots, and blend together in the nutribullet. This is an appropriate meal for 6-month olds since they are unable to chew food.

Chapter 14

Water (No Substitute)

Years ago, I remember a colleague discussing with me a topic aired on either Dateline or a similar show. It was discussed whether or not a person could drink fluids other than water and still receive the same nutritional benefits or proper nourishment as if they had only consumed water. This was back then when the recommended daily amount of water was 64 ounces or 8 eight-ounce glasses of water instead of what it is today. This colleague informed me that the expert(s) suggested it was okay to even drink conventional fruit juices at grocery stores in place of water. Back then they did not understand the importance of limiting sugar intake. Most conventional juices and even some organic juices are filled with a bunch of sugar. If there was any nutritional value in the fruits from which these juices were derived, it has probably been diminished due to processing.

Our bodies are at least 60% percent water. Experts recommend you drink at least half of your body weight in ounces. As discussed in Chapter 14: Vegetables and Fruits, you may be required to drink more water contingent upon your level of activity and whether or not you live in a warmer or cooler climate. Warmer climates typically require more hydration. A helpful tip is to drink more water at room temperature. People tend to drink less water when the water is cold as opposed to when it is warm.

I personally do not drink tap water. I drink only bottled water. I personally do not consume tap water unless I shower, brush my teeth, or wash my hands. If I am able to do so, I cook with bottled water. When I am able to afford water and air purifiers, I intend to purchase them. Being a resident of Michigan and the whole "Flint water crisis", I am sure you can understand my perspective. The water department does not completely filter the water of all toxins. They allow "acceptable levels" of lead and other toxins in public drinking water.

Water is not just a nutritional issue, but also an environmental issue. As bright as the scientific mind are of this country and around all the world and all of the technological advancement, I do not understand how parts of this country, especially California, can have a water shortage despite being surrounded by massive bodies of water.

There are several different types of bottled water to choose from:

1. Alkaline water:

   Alkaline Water is water that has a pH greater than 7.0. Alkaline refers to pH. pH is a number that measures how acidic or alkaline a substance is on a scale of 0 to 14. Example: A pH of 1 would be very acidic. A pH of 13 would be very alkaline. <u>Alkaline water can either be natural or purified</u> water with minerals added. Natural alkaline water contains a higher pH by dissolving earth's natural underground minerals from porous rocks. Other alkaline waters are purified water with minerals added. They use a chemical process like electrolysis to split water molecules apart with electricity to artificially create a higher pH in the water.

2. Purified water:

   Purified water is any type of water that has been treated with an action to "purify" it. The water is purified to remove any chemicals or contaminants that may be present. The types of purification include distillation, deionization, reverse osmosis and carbon filtration. Some bottling facilities add a light blend of minerals back into the water after the purification process in order to give the water taste.

3. Distilled water:

   Distilled water is water that goes through a purification process called distillation. This process replicates the earth's natural hydrological cycle and boils away impurities while capturing only H_2O, resulting in water that is in its purest chemical form. <u>Distilled water has many more uses</u> than just drinking water. Many know distilled water for its uses in medical equipment, humidifiers and automobiles due to its complete absence of mineral content.

4. Spring water:

Spring water according to the <u>U.S. Food & Drug Administration</u> (FDA) is "water derived from an underground formation from which water flows naturally to the surface of the earth at an identified location." A spring forms when an underground aquifer is filled and the excess seeps through to the surface. <u>Bottled spring water is gathered at the source</u> and transported to a bottling facility where it is treated and tested to meet all FDA standards and requirements.

Some water bottles may contain bisphenol A or BPA. Bisphenol A, or BPA, is a chemical used to make a hard clear plastic called polycarbonate, some sealants, and thermal paper such as the paper used to print cash register receipts. Some experts recommend plastic containers labeled with a 1, 2, 4, or 5. These experts also advise you to avoid plastic containers labeled 3, 6, and most plastics labelled 7.

Water is definitely a much healthier beverage alternative for you as opposed to soda, energy drinks, and carbonated beverages. Energy drinks was discussed in Chapter 3: No Meats, Limited Sugar, and No Caffeine. Needless to say, carbonated beverages inclusive of alcohol and sodas are not good for you either. Throughout the earlier chapters of this book, you were advised not to consume alcohol for various reasons. A healthy alternative to unhealthy beverages such as sodas, processed sugary drinks, carbonated beverages, and alcohol are organic or natural decaffeinated green and herbal teas. You can find these types of teas in a lot of grocery stores nationwide in their tea aisle.

However, you should still drink water.

Benefits of drinking water:

1. Increased energy
2. Flushes out toxins
3. Energizes muscles
4. Regulates body temperature
5. Increases dental health
6. Aids in food digestion
7. Promotes weight loss
8. Provides glowing skin
9. Lubricates joints

Sources

Chapter 2: No Meat, Limited Sugar, No Caffeine

1. Sollid, K. (2014 May 23). "Questions and Answers About Sugars". *International Food Information Council Foundation.* (2018 November 8). https://www.foodinsight.org/Questions and Answers About Sugars

2. Josh, A. (2016 October 31). "Why You Should Avoid Pork". *Draxe.com.* (2018 November 8). https://draxe.com/why-you-should-avoid-pork/.

3. Kravitz, M. (2017 March 1). "Organic meat vs non-organic meat" What does paying more really buy you?". *Mic.* (2018 November 8). https://mic.com/articles/168052/organic-meat-vs-non-organic-meat-what-does-paying-more-really-buy-you#KHwTMbp9x.

4. Gunnars, K. (2018 May 22). "Is Red Meat Bad for You, or Good? An Objective Look". *Healthline.com.* (2018 November 8). https://www.healthline.com/nutrition/is-red-meat-bad-for-you-or-good.

5. Dickinson, K. Bernstein, J. (2018 March 7). "If sugar is so bad for us, why is the sugar in fruit ok?". *The Conversation.* (2018 November 8). theconversation.com/if-sugar-is-so-bad-for-us-why-is-the-sugar-in-fruit-ok-89958.

6. Braft, D. (2018 July 30). "I'm a Size 2, buy My Cholesterol Was Approaching Stroke Levels". *Healthline.com.* (2018 November 8). https://www.healthline.com/health/cholesterol/skinny-but-high-cholesterol.

7. Organic Consumers Association. (2007 May 1). "Growth Hormones Fed to Beef Cattle Damage Human Health". (2018 November 8). https://www.organicconsumers.org/scientific/growth-hormones-fed-beef-cattle-damage-human-health.

8. The Society for Cardiovascular Angiography and Interventions. (2015 January 1). "Energy Drinks & The Heart: Know the Risks". *SecondsCount.* (2018 November 8). www.secondscount.org/heart-condition-centers/info-detail-2/energy-drinks--heart-know-risks#.XDfpH1xKiUk.

9. Kashubara, K. (2017 August 14). "Difference Between Triglycerides & Cholesterol". *Livestrong.com.* (2018 November 8). https://www.livestrong.com/article/112746-difference-between-triglycerides-cholesterol/.

10. The Vegan Society. "Definition of Veganism". (2018 November 8). https://www.vegansociety.com/go-vegan/definition-veganism.

11. Chait, J. (2018 October 22). "What Does Free Range Really Mean?". (2018 November 8). https://www.thebalancesmb.com/what-does-free-range-really-mean-2538247.

12. Gunnars, K. (2018 June 28). "Daily Intake of Sugar – How Much Sugar Should You Eat Per Day?". *Healthline.com.* (2018 November 8). https://healthline.com/nutrition/how-much-sugar-per-day.

13. Perry, S. (2014 March 6). "Cut sugar consumption to 5 percent of total daily calories, experts say". (2018 November 8). https://www.minnpost.com/second-opinion/2014/03/cut-sugar-consumption-5-percent-total-daily-calories-experts-say/.

14. Kim, Y. Chang, H. (June 2011). "Correlation between attention deficit hyperactivity disorder and sugar consumption, quality of diet, and dietary behavior in school children". *Nutrition Research and Practice.* (2018 November 8). https://www.ncbi.nlm.nih.gov/pmc/articles/PMC3133757/.

15. Schaefer, A. MCDermott, A. ed. Laflamme, M. (2016 March 29). "Coffee and Cholesterol: Is there a link?" *Healthline.com.* (2018 November 8). https://www.healthline.com/health/high-cholesterol/coffee-link.

16. Medline Plus. (2018 October 23). "Cholesterol". (2018 November 8). https://medlineplus.gov/cholesterol.html.

17. National Health Service. (2011 November 4). "Cancer risk of overcooked meat tested in mice". (2018 November 8). https://www.nhs.uk/news/cancer/cancer-risk-of-overcooked-meat-tested-in-mice/.

18. Mayo Foundation for Medical Education and Research. (2017 March 8). "Caffeine: How much is too much?". *Mayoclinic.org.* (2018 November 8). https://www.mayoclinic.org/healthy-lifestyle/nutrition-and-healthy-eating/in-depth/caffeine/art-20045678.

19. Blood Pressure UK. "Why salt is bad". (2018 November 8). www.bloodpressureuk.org/microsites/salt/Home/Whysaltisbad.

20. Helpguide.com. (2018 December 14). "ADHD in Children Recognizing the Signs and Symptoms and Getting Help". (2018 December 14). https://www.helpguide.org/articles/add-adhd/attention-deficit-disorder-adhd-in-children.htm/.

21. Additude Editors. "Why Sugar is Kryptonite for ADHD Brains". *Additude Mag.* (2018 November 8). https://www.additudemag.com/adhd-diet-nutrition-sugar.

22. Meat Poultry Nutrition Organization. "12 Good Reasons Meat and Poultry Should be Part of Your Balanced Diet". (2018 November 8). www.meatpoultrynutrition.org/content/great-taste-alone-shouldnt-dictate-your-dietary-choices-here-are-12-good-reasons-meat-and.

23. Hyman, M. "10 Reasons to Quit Coffee (Plus Healthy Alternatives). (2018 November 8). www.hungryforchange.tv/article/10-reasons-to-quit-coffee-plus-healthy-alternatives.

24. The Ecology Center. (2016 August 25). "10 Reasons to Eat Grass-Fed & Cage-Free Meat". (2018 November 8). https://www.theecologycenter.org/resources/10-reasons-to-eat-grass-fed-cage-free-meat/.

25. Patel, A. (2018 January 27). "The healthiest ways to cook your favourite meat". *Global News*. (2018 November 8). https://globalnews.ca/news/3987387/healthy-ways-cook-meat/.

26. Gardner, A. "9 Foods Additives That May Affect ADHD". (2018 November 8). https://www.health.com/adhd/9-food-additives-that-may-affect-adhd.

27. The Salt Association. "Salt & The Function of Our Cells". (2018 November 8). https://www.saltassociation.co.uk/education/salt-health/salt-function-cells/.

28. Wikipedia.com. (2018 September 25). "Starch". (2018 November 8). https://en.wikipedia.org/wiki/Starch.

29. Nutritionandyou.com. "Stevia plant (herb) nutrition facts". (2018 November 8). https://www.nutrition-and-you.com/stevia-plant.html.

30. National Kidney Foundation. "Sugar and Your Kidneys". (2018 November 8). https://www.kidney.org/content/sugar-and-your-kidneys.

31. Sheehan, J. "The Advantages of Broiling Food". *Healthy Eating | SF GATE*. (2018 December 8). https://healthyeating.sfgate.com/advantages-broiling-food-7766.html.

32. Wayne, M. "The Meat You Eat: Steroid Use in Livestock". (2018 December 8). https://drmichaelwayne.com/blog/the-meat-you-eat-steroid-use-in-livestock/.

33. Cespedes, A. "The Nutrition of Melted Cheese". *Our Everyday Life.* (2018 December 8). https://oureverydaylife.com/333832-the-nutrition-of-melted-cheese.html.

34. Kallmyer, T. (2018 November 11). "Top 15 + Energy Drink Dangers". *Caffeine Informer*. (2018 December 8). https://www.caffeineinformer.com/top-10-energy-drink-dangers.

35. Hoffman, M. ed. Smith, M. (updated 2018 December 18). "Safer Food For a Healthier You". *Web MD*. (2018 December 8). https://www.webmd.com/diet/features/safer-food-healthier-you#1.

36. Dr. Edward Group. (2015 December 4). "Vegan vs. Vegetarian: Differences and Similarities". (2018 December 8)). https://www.globalhealingcenter.com/natural-health/vegan-vs-vegetarian/.

37. Bazian. National Health Service. (2014 October 15). "Warnings issued over energy drinks". (2018 December 8). https://www.nhs.uk/news/food-and-diet/warnings-issued-over-energy-drinks/.

38. Norton, A. (2018 March 18). "Well-Done Meat Not Good for Your Blood Pressure". *Web MD*. (2018 December 8). https://www.webmd.com/food-recipes/news/20180321/well-done-meat-not-good-for-your-blood-pressure#1.

39. Cox, L. (2018 April 26). "What Is Stevia?" *Live Science*. (2018 December 8). https://www.livescience.com/39601-stevia-facts-safety.html.

40. Renee, J. (2018 November 21). "What Is the Importance of Water & Salt in Body Homeostasis?". *Healthy Eating | SF Gate*. (2018 December 8). https://healthyeating.sfgate.com/importance-water-salt-body-homeostasis-10409.html.

41. Dolson, L. (2018 November 7). "Why Do Potatoes Have a Higher Glycemic Index Than Sugar?". *Very Well Fit*. (2018 December 8). https://www.verywellfit.com/why-do-potatoes-raise-blood-glucose-more-than-sugar-2242317..

42. Matthews, M. (2014 April 23). "You'll Stop Worrying About Sugar After Reading This Article". (2018 December 8). Https://www.muscleforlife.com/sugar-facts/.

43. Sindelar, J. (2012 October 18). "What's the Deal with Nitrates and Nitrites Used in Meat Products?" (2018 December 8). https://fyi.extension.wisc.edu/meats/files/2012/02/Nitrate-and-nitrite-in-cured-meat_10-18-2012.pdf.

Chapter 5: Natural then Mostly Organic

1. Sholl, J. (October 2011). "8 Hidden Toxins: What's Lurking in Your Cleaning Products?". *Experience Life*. (2018 December 9). https://experiencelife.com/article/8-hidden-toxins-whats-lurking-in-your-cleaning-products/.

2. Colquhoun, J. (2016 November 1). "22 Additives And Preservatives To Avoid". *Food Matters*. (2018 December 9). https://www.foodmatters.com/article/22-additives-and-preservatives-to-avoid.

3. DeCostole, J. (2017 November 29). "5 Things You Should Know About Organic". *Redbookmag.com*. (2018 December 9). https://www.redbookmag.com/body/healthy-eating/a2016/truth-about-organic-foods/.

4. Butler, T. "How Does Organic Food Affect Your Body". *Love to Know Home & Garden*. (2018 December 9). https://organic.lovetoknow.com/How_Does_Organic_Food_Affect_Your_Body.

5. United States Department of Agriculture. "Organic Labeling Standards". (2018 December 9). https://www.ams.usda.gov/grades-standards/organic-labeling-standards.

Chapter 6: Organic and Natural Supplements

1. Medline Plus. (2018 July 13). "Minerals". (2018 December 10). https://medlineplus.gov/minerals.html.

2. Ed. Romito, K. and O'brien, R. (2018 March 28). "Minerals: Their Functions and Sources". *Michigan Medicine University of Michigan.* (2018 December 10). https://www.uofmhealth.org/health-library/ta3912.

3. National Center for Biotechnology Information. "Muscle and Bones". (2018 November 7). https://www.ncbi.nlm.nih.gov/books/NBK22228/.

4. ed. Ratini, M. (2018 June 19). "Vitamins and Minerals: How much should you take?". *Web MD.* (2018 December 12). https://www.webmd.com/vitamins-and-supplements/vitamins-minerals-how-much-should-you-take#1.

5. Harvard Health Letter. (May 2015). "Should you get your nutrients from food or from supplements?". *Harvard Medical School.* (2018 December 10). https://www.health.harvard.edu/staying-healthy/should-you-get-your-nutrients-from-food-or-from-supplements.

6. Turner, L. (2018 March 12). "The Best Time of the Day to Take 7 Popular Supplements". *The Vitamin Shoppe.* (2018 December 10). https://whatsgood.vitaminshoppe.com/supplement-timing/.

7. Fletcher, J. ed. Wilson, D. (2017 September 28). "When is the best time to take vitamins?". *Medical News Today.* (2018 December 10). https//www.medicalnewstoday.com/articles/319556.php.

8. Lenntech.com. "Recommended daily intake of vitamins and minerals". (2018 December 12). https://www.lenntech.com/recommended-daily-intake.htm.

9. Myprotein.com. (2016 January 21). "Supplement Timing/ With Food or An Empty Stomach?" (2018 December 10). https://us.myprotein.com/thezone/supplements/supplement-timing-empty-stomach/.

10. Mamavation.com. "Toxic Vitamins: How to Pick a Supplement that's Clean for Your Family". (2018 December 12). https://www.mamavation.com/featured/toxic-vitamins-how-to-pick-a-supplement-thats-clean-for-your-family.html.

11. Better Health Channel Victoria State Government. (September 2012). "Vitamins – common misconceptions". (2018 December 10).

https://www.betterhealth.vic.gov.au/health/healthyliving/vitamins-common-misconceptions.

12. Medline Plus. (2018 July 13). "Vitamins". (2018 December 10). https://medlineplus.gov/vitamins.html.

13. Natural Balance Foods. "What are Macronutrients & Micronutrients?" (2012 December 12). https://www.naturalbalancefoods.com/community/dietary-needs/what-are-macronutrients-micronutrients/.

14. Study.com. (2015 October 26). "What are Micronutrients? - Definition, Types, Foods & Importance". (2018 December 12). https://study.com/academy/lesson/what-are-micronutrients-definition-types-foods-importance.html.

15. Study.com. (2015 August 31). "What are vitamins? - Definition, Types, Purpose & Examples". (2018 December 10). https://study.com/academy/lesson/what-are-vitamins-definition-types-purpose-examples.html.

16. The Organic & Non-GMO Report. "What is Non-GMO? What are genetically modified foods?" (2018 December 12). non-gmoreport.com/what-is-non-gmo-what-are-genetically-modified-foods/.

17. White, R. (2018 June 5). "7 Essential Nutrients Your Body Needs". *Wellness Daily*. (2018 December 12). https://www.wellnessdaily.com.au/health/7-essential-nutrients-your-body-needs.

18. Schaefer, A. (2015 May 21). "10 Things That Happen When You Sit Down All Day". *Healthline.com*. (2018 November 8). https://www.healthline.com/health/workplace-health/things-that-happen-when-you-sit-down-all-day#1.

19. Nursingdegree.net. "100 Best Herbs for Your Health and Wellness". (2018 December 10). www.nursingdegree.net/blog/32/100-best-herbs-for-your-health-and-wellness/.

20. Medline Plus. (2015 February 9). "Definitions of Health Terms: Minerals". (2018 December 10). https://medlineplus.gov/definitions/mineralsdefinitions.html.

21. Wikipedia.com. (updated 2019 January 10). "Herb". (2018 December 10). https://en.wikipedia.org/wiki/Herb.

22. Amir, S. (2015 August 24). "How Long Does It Take Supplements to Work?". *Nutrition Sheila*. (2018 December 12).

https://www.nutritionsheila.com/nutrition-applied-blog/how-long-does-it-take-supplements-to-work.

23. Amir, S. (2018 September 1). "Here's How Long It Actually Takes For a Supplement to Kick In". *Elite Daily.* (2018 December 12). https://www.elitedaily.com/wellness/how-long-takes-supplement-kick-in/1542896.

24. John Hopkins Medical Organization. "Is There Really Any Benefit to Multi-vitamins?". (2018 December 10). https://www.hopkinsmedicine.org/health/healthy_aging/healthy_body/is-there-really-any-benefit-to-multivitamins.

25. Seattle Organic Restaurants. "List of top 10 toxic chemicals, preservatives and harmful additives in supplements and foods". (2018 December 12). www.seattleorganicrestaurants.com/vegan-whole-food/toxic-chemicals-gmo-ingredients-in-nutritional-supplements.php.

26. Harvard Medical School. (2017 August 14). "Listing of Vitamins". (2018 December 10). https://www.health.harvard.edu/staying-healthy/listing of vitamins

27. Chandler, S. (2018 April 3). "Minerals That a Human Body Needs". *Healthy Eating | SF Gate.* (2018 December 10). https://healthyeating.sfgate.com/minerals-human-body-needs-5555.html.

28. Buckley, D. (2018 February 15). "6 Harmful Additives that Could be Lurking in Your Supplements". *Natural Stacks.* (2018 December 12). https://www.naturalstacks.com/blogs/news/6-harmful-supplement-additives.

29. Yigzaw, E. (2016 December 2). "5 Dangerous Ingredients in Your Vitamins and Dietary Supplements". *American College of Healthcare Sciences.* (2018 December 12). info.achs.edu/blog/5-dangerous-ingredients-in-your-vitamins-and-dietary-supplements.

1. Borreli, L. (2013 August 10). "Microwaves Are Bad For You: 5 Reasons Why Microwave Oven Cooking Is Harming Your Health". *Medical Daily.* (2018 December 10). https://www.medicaldaily.com/microwaves-are-bad-you-5-reasons-why-microwave-oven-cooking-harming-your-health-250145.

Chapter 9: Gluten-Free, Soy-Free, and Reduced Fried Foods

1. Jaarin, K. Kamsiah, Y. (2012 August 29). "Repeatedly Heated Vegetable Oils and Lipid Peroxidation". (2018 December 15). https://www.intechopen.com/books/lipid-peroxidation/repeatedly-heated-vegetable-oils-and-lipid-peroxidation.

2. Prahran Market. (2016 August 26). "5 Different Ways to Fry". (2018 December 15). https://www.prahanmarket.com/au/5-different-ways-to-fry/.

3. Ducharme, J. (2017 October 25). "5 Things That happen to Your Body When You Eat Greasy Food". *Time.* (2018 December 15). time.com/4996776/greasy-food-bad-for-you/.

4. Gunnars, K. (2013 November 11). "6 Reasons Why Gluten Is Bad for Some People". *Healthline.com.* (2018 December 14). https://www.healthline.com/nutrition/6-shocking-reasons-why-gluten-is-bad.

5. Hotze Health. (2018 August 1). "7 Reasons Gluten Is Bad for Your Brain". *Hotze Health & Wellness Center.* (2018 December 14). https://www.hotzehwc.com/2018/08/7-reasons-gluten-is-bad-for-your-brain/.

6. Paleoleap.com. "11 Ways Gluten and Wheat can Damage Your Health". (2018 December 14). https://paleoleap.com/11-ways-gluten-and-wheat-can-damage-your-health/.

7. Holly, W. (2014 January 14). "A Vegan Doctor Addresses Soy Myths and Misinformation". *Free From Harm.* (2018 December 15). https//freefromharm.org/health-nutrition/vegan-doctor-addresses-soy-myths-and-misinformation/.

8. American Nutrition Association. "The Whole Soy Story". *Nutrition Digest.* (2018 December 15). americannutritionassociation.org/newsletter/whole-soy-story

9. Burkhart, A. (March 2015). "Arsenic in Rice & The Gluten Free Diet: Facts and Tips". (2018 December 14). theceliacmd.com/2015/03/arsenic-in-rice-the-gluten-free-diet-facts-and-tips/.

10. Oberst, L. (2018 March 2). "Arsenic in Rice: How Concerned Should You Be?". *Food Revolution Network.* (2018 December 15). https://foodrevolution.org/blog/arsenic-in-rice/.

11. San Diego Fertility Center. (2005 January 1). "Does Soy Cause Infertility?". *San Diego Fertility Center Miracle B90log.* (2018 December 15). https://www.sdfertility.com/blog/does-soy-cause-infertility#.

12. Dr. Helmenstine. (2018 November 29). "What is Gluten? Chemistry and Food Sources". *Thoughtco.com.* (2018 December 14). https://www.thoughtco.com/gluten-chemistry-and-food-sources-607388.

13. Canadian Grain Commission. (2016 March 29). "Gluten's role in bread baking performance". (2018 December 14). https://www.grainscanada.gc.ca/fact-fait/gluten-eng.htm.

14. Chun-Yi, N. Xin_Fang, L. Norliana, M. Siti, A. Yusof, K. Kamisiah, J. "Heated vegetable oils and cardiovascular disease risk factors". *Vascular Pharmacology Volume 61, Issue 1, Pages 1-9.* (2018 December 14. https://www.sciencedirect.com/science/article/pii/S1537189114000536.

15. Watson, S. ed. Nazario, B. (2017 June 22). "How Bad for You Are Fried Foods?" *Web MD.* (2018 December 15). https://www.webmd.com/diet/news/20170622/how-bad-for-you-are-fried-foods.

16. Mercola, J. "How to Get the Benefits of Soy without All the Health Risks". *Mercola.* (2018 December 15). https://www.mercola.com/Downloads/bonus/dangers-of-soy/report.aspx.

17. Groves, M. (2018 November 22). "Is Soy Good or Bad for your Health?" *Healthline.com.* (2018 December 15). https://www.healthline.com/nutrition/soy-good-or-bad.

18. Dellitt, J. "Let's Break Down the Benefits and Risks of Soy". *Aaptiv.* (2018 December 15). https://aaptiv.com/magazine/benefits-and-risks-of-soy.

19. Foodbabe.com. "Processed To Death – Get These Cooking Oils Out of Your Pantry STAT!". (2018 December 15). https://foodbabe.com/cooking-oils/.

20. Cleveland Clinic. (December 2013). "Soy Foods: Benefits of Soy". (2018 December 15). https://my.clevelandclinic.org/health/articles/17491-soy-foods/benefits-of-soy.

21. Schwartz, S. (2015 November 8). "The 5 Worst Foods For Your Brain". *Huff Post.* (2018 December 15). https://www.huffingtonpost.com/entry/the-5-worst-foods-for-your-brain_us_563d1713e4b0411d30711ac4.

22. Fitzsimmons, K. (2013 February 25). "The Danger of Cooking with Healthy Oils Past Their Smoke Point". (2018 December 15).

https://www.business2community.com/health-wellness/the-danger-of-cooking-wth-healthy-oils-past-their-smoke-point-0418150.

23. Naturalhealthstrategies.com. "The Dangers of Soy Are Real – and Much Worse Than You Might Think". (2018 December 15). www.naturalhealthstrategies.com/dangers-of-soy.html.

24. Broaddus, H. (2017 July 17). "The Difference Between Solvent Expelled, Expeller Pressed And Cold Pressed Oil". *Centra Foods.* (2018 December 15). www.centrafoods.com/blog/the-difference-between-solvent-expelled-expeller-pressed-and-cold-pressed-oil.

25. Fharzana. (2012 January 12). "The Science Behind Cooking With Oil". *Chowhound.* (2018 December 15). https://www.chowhound.com/post/science-cooking-oil-827996.

26. Barrett, J. (June 2006). "The Science of Soy: What Do We Really Know?". *Environmental Health Perspectives.* (2018 December 15). https://www.ncbi.nlm.nih.gov/pmc/PMC1480510/.

27. Celiac Disease Foundation. "What is Gluten?". (2018 December 14). https://celiac.org/gluten-free-living/what-is-gluten/.

28. Specter, M. (2014 November 3). "Against the Grain". *The New Yorker.* (2018 December 14). https://www.newyorker.com/magazine/2014/11/03/grain.

29. The Cooking Science Guy. (July 2012). "Explaining Gluten". (2018 December 14). www.cookingscienceguy.com/pages/wp-content/uploads/2012/07/Explaining-Gluten.pdf

Chapter 10: No Fried Food

1. American Cancer Society. (2016 March 10). "Acrylamide and Cancer Risk". (2018 December 15). https://www.cancer.org/cancer/cancer-causes/acrylamide.html.

2. Gunnars, K. (2017 June 4). "Are Nitrates and Nitrites in Foods Harmful?" *Healthline.com.* (2018 Dec. 8). https://www.healthline.com/nutrition/are-nitrates-and-nitrites-harmful.

3. Good, J. (2012 April 17). "Healthiest cooking oil comparison chart with smoke points and omega 3 fatty acid ratios". *The Baseline of Health Foundation.* (2018 December 15). https://jonbarron.org/diet-and-nutrition/healthiest-cooking-oil-chart-smoke-points.

4. Fitzsimmons, K. (2013 February 25). "The Danger of Cooking with Healthy Oils Past Their Smoke Point". (2018 December 15). https://www.business2community.com/health-wellness/the-danger-of-cooking-wth-healthy-oils-past-their-smoke-point-0418150.

Chapter 11: 6:00 a.m. – 6:00 p.m.

1. Gunnars, K. (2017 June 4). "6 Popular Ways to Do Intermittent Fasting". *Healthline.com.* (2018 December 15). https://www.healthline.com/nutrition/6-ways-to-do-intermittent-fasting.
2. Gunnars, K. (2016 August 16). "10 Evidence-Based Health Benefits of Intermittent Fasting". *Healthline.com.* (2018 December 15). https://www.healthline.com/nutrition/10-health-benefits-of-intermittent-fasting.
3. Fung, J. (2018 December 10). "Intermittent fasting for beginners". *Dietdoctor.com.* (2018 December 15). https://www.dietdoctor.com/intermittent-fasting.
4. Mukherjee, T. (2018 December 13). "What Is Intermittent Fasting, and Does It Help You Lose Weight?" *Prevention.* (2018 December 15). https://www.prevention.com/weight-loss/a20500235/intermittent-fasting/.

1. Wells, K. (2018 July 15). "Why Saturated Fat Is Not the Enemy (& Why We Need It)." *Wellness Mama.* (2018 December 22). https://wellnessmama.com/1265/saturated-fat/.

2. Pope, S. "When Omega-3 Fats Can Be Dangerous to Your Health". *The Health Economist.* (2018 December 22). https://www.thehealthyhomeeconomist.com/when-omega-3-fats-can-be-dangerous-to-your-health/.

3. Floraproactive.co.uk. "What are Saturated and Unsaturated Fats?" (2018 December 22). https://floraproactive.co.uk/what-is-cholesterol/saturated-and-unsaturated-fats/what-are-saturated-and-unsaturated-fats/.

4. Novak, S. (2014 March 12). "Unsaturated Fat Overload: Can You Eat Too Many Good Fats?". *Organic Authority.* https://www.organicauthority.com/health/unsaturated-fat-overload-can-you-eat-too-many-good-fats.

5. Weil, A. (2012 January 27). "Too Much Omega-3?" (2018 December 22). https://www.drweil.com/vitamins-supplements-herbs/vitamins/too-much-omega-3/.

6. Moll, J. (2018 October 15). "The Difference Between Saturated and Unsaturated Fats". *verywellhealth.com.* (2018 December 22). https://www.verywellhealth.com/difference-between-saturated-fats-and-unsaturated-fats-697517.

7. Webber, L. "Side Effects of Omega 3-6-9". *Livestrong.com.* (2018 December 22). https://www.livestrong.com/article/336486-side-effects-of-omega-3-6-9/.

8. Wikipedia.com. (2018 December 14). "Saturated Fat". (2018 December 22). https://en.wikipedia.org/wiki/Saturated_fat.

9. Cooley, J. (2018 July 16). "Know Your Fats: Balancing the Omega 3 6 9 Ratio". *University Health News Daily.* (2018 December 22). https://universityhealthnews.com/daily/nutrition/know-your-fats-balancing-3-6-9-omega-ratio/.

10. Weisenberg, J. (September 2013). "Heart – Healthy Fats – It's The Type – Not – The Amount – That – Matters". *Today's Dietitian Volume 15 No.9 Page 14.* (2018 December 22). https://todaysdietitian.com/newarchives/090313p14.shtml.

11. Mayo Foundation for Medical Education and Research. "Fish Oil". (2018 December 22). https://www.mayoclinic.org/drugs-supplements-fish-oil/art-20364810.

12. Medline Plus. (2018 December 6). "Facts About Saturated Fats". (2018 December 22). https://medlineplus.gov/ency/patientinstructions/000838.htm.

13. Medline Plus. (2018 December 6). "Facts about polyunsaturated fats". (2018 December 22). https://medlineplus.gov/ency/patientinstructions/000747.htm.

14. Medicine Net. (2016 May 13). "Medical Definition of Trans Fat". (2018 December 22). https://www.medicinenet.com/script/main/art.asp?articlekey=11091.

15. Medicine Net. (2018 December 11). "Medical Definition of Saturated Fat". (2018 December 22). https://www.medicinenet.com/script/main/art.asp?articlekey=18388.

16. Basch, L. "Can You Eat Too Much Healthy Fat? A Registered Dietitian Explains". *mindbodygreens.com.* (2018 December 22). https://www.mindbodygreen.com/0-23747/can-you-eat-too-much-healthy-fat-a-registered-dietitian-explains.html.

17. Link, R. (2018 July 17). "8 Little – Known Side Effects of Too Much Fish Oil". *Healthline.com.* (2018 December 22). https://www.healthline.com/nutrition/fish-oil-side-effects.

18. American Heart Association. (2017 March 23). "Trans Fats". (2018 December 22). https://www.heart.org/en/healthy-living/healthy-eating/eat-smart/facts/trans-fat.

Chapter 13: Vegetables and Fruits

1. Anu Rahal, Mahima , Amit Kumar Verma, Amit Kumar , Ruchi Tiwari , Sanjay Kapoor , Sandip Chakraborty and Kuldeep Dhama (2014 January 11). Phytonutrients and Nutraceuticals in Vegetables and Their Multi-dimensional Medicinal and Health Benefits for Humans and Their Companion Animals: A Review. *Journal of Biological Sciences, 14: 1-19.* DOI: 10.3923/jbs.2014.1.19 URL: https://scialert.net/abstract/?doi=jbs.2014.1.19.

2. Dr. Jockers. "12 Herbs That Kill Parasites Naturally". (2018 December 22). https://drjockers.com/12-herbs-kill-parasites-naturally/.

3. Fruitsandveggiematters.org. "About The Buzz: Frozen and Canned Fruits and Vegetables vs Fresh". (2018 December 22). https://www.fruitsandveggiesmorematters.org/frozen-and-canned-fruits-and-vegetables-vs-fresh.

4. Rabin, R.C. (2016 November 18). "Are Frozen Fruits and Vegetables as Nutritious as Fresh?" *Blog New York Times.* (2018 December 22). https://well.blogs.nytimes.com/2016/11/18/are-frozen-fruits-abd-vegetables-nutritious-as-fresh/.

5. Liu, D. (2015 November 22). "How does the stomach handle liquid vs. solid food?" *Medical Sciences Stack Exchange.* (2018 December 22). https://medicalsciences.stackexchange.com/questions/3668/how-does-the-stomach-handle-liquid-vs-solid-food.

6. Davidson, J. (2017 March 28). "Don't Feed The Parasite: Best Natural Cleanse Solutions". (2018 December 22). https://drjaydavidson.com/dont-feed-parasites/.

7. American Heart Association. (2018). "Fruits and Vegetables Serving Sizes". (2018 December 22). https://www.heart.org/en/healthy-living/healthy-eating/add-color/fruits-and-vegetables-serving-sizes.

8. Walters, C. Original Vitamix Dealer. (2014 June 25). "How long will my smoothie last for in the fridge?". *Raw Blend.* (2018 December 22). https://www.rawblend.com.au/blog/how-long-will-my-smoothie-last-for-in-the-fridge/.

9. Shaw, G. ed. Nazario, B. (2009 July 7). "Water and Your Diet: Staying Slim and Regular with H20". *Web MD*. (2018 December 22). https://www.webmd.com/diet/features/water-for-weight-loss/diet#1.

10. Goaskalice.com. (2017 November 10). "Nutritional Differences between Canned, Frozen, and Fresh Veggies?". (2018 December 22). https://goaskalice.columbia.edu/answered-questions/nutritional-differences-between-canned-frozen-and-fresh-veggies-0.

11. Berardi, J. "Soil depletion and organic produce". *Precision Nutrition*. (2018 December 22). https://www.precisionnutrition.com/soil-depletion-organic-produce.

12. Sachdev, I.(2018 January 15). "Easy Tips to Wash Your Fruits And Vegetables". *Sepalika.* (2018 December 22). https://www.sepalika.com/living-well/washing-fruits-and-vegetables/.

13. Karthik. (2018 June 11). "Why does a farmer rotate crops in the field?". *Quora.com.* (2018 December 9). https://www.quora.com/Why-does-a-farmer-rotate-crops-in-the-fields.

Chapter 14: Water (No Substitute)

1. Shaw, G. ed. Nazario, B. (2009 July 7). *"Water and Your Diet: Staying Slim and Regular with H20"*. Web MD. (2018 December 22). https://www.webmd.com/diet/features/water-for-weight-loss-diet#1.

2. The Water Guy. *"What is the difference in bottled water types"*. (2018 December 23). https://www.waterguys.com/blog/bottled-water-types/.

3. Hellonaturalliving.com. (2016 February 18). *"Are any of the #7 plastics safe?"*. (2019 January 13). https://www.hellonaturalliving.com/are-any-of-the-7-plastics-safe/.

4. Sierra Club Michigan Chapter. *"BPA"*. (2019 January 13). https://www.sierraclub.org/michigan/bpa.

www.ingramcontent.com/pod-product-compliance
Lightning Source LLC
Chambersburg PA
CBHW081934160726
47999CB00008B/2386